Examining the Use of Biomarkers in Establishing the Presence and Severity of Impairments

PROCEEDINGS OF A WORKSHOP

Megan Snair, Tracy A. Lustig, and Cyndi Trang, *Rapporteurs*

Board on Health Care Services

Health and Medicine Division

The National Academies of
SCIENCES · ENGINEERING · MEDICINE

THE NATIONAL ACADEMIES PRESS
Washington, DC
www.nap.edu

THE NATIONAL ACADEMIES PRESS 500 Fifth Street, NW Washington, DC 20001

This activity was supported by a contract between the National Academy of Sciences and the Social Security Administration. Any opinions, findings, conclusions, or recommendations expressed in this publication do not necessarily reflect the views of any organization or agency that provided support for the project.

International Standard Book Number-13: 978-0-309-68263-3
International Standard Book Number-10: 0-309-68263-0
Digital Object Identifier: https://doi.org/10.17226/25926

Additional copies of this publication are available from the National Academies Press, 500 Fifth Street, NW, Keck 360, Washington, DC 20001; (800) 624-6242 or (202) 334-3313; http://www.nap.edu.

Copyright 2020 by the National Academy of Sciences. All rights reserved.

Printed in the United States of America

Suggested citation: National Academies of Sciences, Engineering, and Medicine. 2020. *Examining the use of biomarkers in establishing the presence and severity of impairments: Proceedings of a workshop.* Washington, DC: The National Academies Press. https://doi.org/10.17226/25926.

The National Academies of
SCIENCES · ENGINEERING · MEDICINE

The **National Academy of Sciences** was established in 1863 by an Act of Congress, signed by President Lincoln, as a private, nongovernmental institution to advise the nation on issues related to science and technology. Members are elected by their peers for outstanding contributions to research. Dr. Marcia McNutt is president.

The **National Academy of Engineering** was established in 1964 under the charter of the National Academy of Sciences to bring the practices of engineering to advising the nation. Members are elected by their peers for extraordinary contributions to engineering. Dr. John L. Anderson is president.

The **National Academy of Medicine** (formerly the Institute of Medicine) was established in 1970 under the charter of the National Academy of Sciences to advise the nation on medical and health issues. Members are elected by their peers for distinguished contributions to medicine and health. Dr. Victor J. Dzau is president.

The three Academies work together as the **National Academies of Sciences, Engineering, and Medicine** to provide independent, objective analysis and advice to the nation and conduct other activities to solve complex problems and inform public policy decisions. The National Academies also encourage education and research, recognize outstanding contributions to knowledge, and increase public understanding in matters of science, engineering, and medicine.

Learn more about the National Academies of Sciences, Engineering, and Medicine at **www.nationalacademies.org**.

The National Academies of
SCIENCES · ENGINEERING · MEDICINE

Consensus Study Reports published by the National Academies of Sciences, Engineering, and Medicine document the evidence-based consensus on the study's statement of task by an authoring committee of experts. Reports typically include findings, conclusions, and recommendations based on information gathered by the committee and the committee's deliberations. Each report has been subjected to a rigorous and independent peer-review process and it represents the position of the National Academies on the statement of task.

Proceedings published by the National Academies of Sciences, Engineering, and Medicine chronicle the presentations and discussions at a workshop, symposium, or other event convened by the National Academies. The statements and opinions contained in proceedings are those of the participants and are not endorsed by other participants, the planning committee, or the National Academies.

For information about other products and activities of the National Academies, please visit www.nationalacademies.org/about/whatwedo.

PLANNING COMMITTEE ON THE STATE OF THE SCIENCE OF THE USE OF BIOMARKERS TO ESTABLISH THE PRESENCE AND SEVERITY OF IMPAIRMENTS[1]

SARA ROSENBAUM (*Chair*), Harold and Jane Hirsh Professor, Health Law and Policy, Milken Institute School of Public Health, The George Washington University
LINDA S. BRADY, Director, Division of Neuroscience and Basic Behavioral Science, National Institute of Mental Health, National Institutes of Health
BETTY DIAMOND, Chief, Autoimmune Disease Center, Feinstein Institutes for Medical Research
SARAH E. MORRIS, Chief, Adult Psychopathology and Psychosocial Intervention Development Branch; Program Officer, Schizophrenia Spectrum Disorders Program, National Institute of Mental Health, National Institutes of Health
RALPH NITKIN, Deputy Director, National Center for Medical Rehabilitation Research; Director, Biological Sciences and Career Development Program, National Institute of Child Health and Human Development, National Institutes of Health
PATRICIA M. OWENS, Consultant, Health and Disability Policy and Programs
SARAH RUIZ, Associate Director, Office of Research Sciences, National Institute on Disability, Independent Living, and Rehabilitation Research
IRA SHOULSON, Professor of Neurology, University of Rochester; Adjunct Professor of Neurology, Georgetown University
ROBERT B. WALLACE, Irene Ensminger Stecher Professor, Cancer Research, The University of Iowa

Health and Medicine Division Staff

TRACY A. LUSTIG, Senior Program Officer
CYNDI TRANG, Research Associate
JOE GOODMAN, Senior Program Assistant
SHARYL NASS, Senior Director, Board on Health Care Services

---

[1] The National Academies of Sciences, Engineering, and Medicine's planning committees are solely responsible for organizing the workshop, identifying topics, and choosing speakers. The responsibility for the published Proceedings of a Workshop rests with the workshop rapporteurs and the institution.

Reviewers

This Proceedings of a Workshop was reviewed in draft form by individuals chosen for their diverse perspectives and technical expertise. The purpose of this independent review is to provide candid and critical comments that will assist the National Academies of Sciences, Engineering, and Medicine in making each published proceedings as sound as possible and to ensure that it meets the institutional standards for quality, objectivity, evidence, and responsiveness to the charge. The review comments and draft manuscript remain confidential to protect the integrity of the process.

We thank the following individuals for their review of this proceedings:

TOM ARRISON, National Academies of Sciences, Engineering, and Medicine
HOWARD H. GOLDMAN, University of Maryland School of Medicine
LAUREN OLIVA, Biogen
MARK RASENICK, University of Illinois College of Medicine

Although the reviewers listed above provided many constructive comments and suggestions, they were not asked to endorse the content of the proceedings nor did they see the final draft before its release. The review of this proceedings was overseen by **WALTER R. FRONTERA,** University of Puerto Rico School of Medicine. He was responsible for making certain that an independent examination of this proceedings was carried out in accordance with standards of the National Academies and that all review comments were carefully considered. Responsibility for the final content rests entirely with the rapporteurs and the National Academies.

Contents

ACRONYMS AND ABBREVIATIONS   xi

1   INTRODUCTION   1
     Background, 2
     Organization of Proceedings, 2

2   UNDERSTANDING BIOMARKER USE AND ITS POTENTIAL FOR DETERMINING HEALTH AND FUNCTION   5
     History and Definition of Biomarkers, 6
     Relating Biomarkers to Health and Function, 9
     Discussion, 13

3   STATE OF THE SCIENCE FOR SPECIFIC IMPAIRMENTS   17
     Major Depression, 18
     Post-Traumatic Stress Disorder, 21
     Schizophrenia, 22
     Chronic Pain and Fibromyalgia, 26
     Arthritis, 28
     Low Back Pain, 31
     Discussion, 33

4	**LEGAL AND ETHICAL IMPLICATIONS**	**37**
	Concerns for the Use of Biomarkers in Disability, 38	
	Potential Harms and Benefits, 39	
	Considerations for Decision Making in Defining Disability, 40	
5	**FINAL THOUGHTS**	**43**
	Examining Positive Findings and Potential Challenges, 44	
	Suggestions for the Use of Biomarkers in the Social Security Administration, 46	

REFERENCES   47

APPENDIXES
A	Statement of Task	53
B	Workshop Agenda	55
C	Biographical Sketches of Workshop Speakers and Planning Committee Members	59

Acronyms and Abbreviations

ACPA	anti-citrullinated peptide antibody
BEST	Biomarkers, EndpointS, and other Tools glossary
CNS	central nervous system
COA	clinical outcome assessment
COU	context of use
EEG	electroencephalogram
FDA	Food and Drug Administration
FNIH	Foundation for the National Institutes of Health
GABA	gamma aminobutyric acid
GPS	global positioning system
HAQ	health assessment questionnaire
ICF	*International Classification of Functioning, Disability and Health*
MRI	magnetic resonance imaging
MVP	Million Veteran Program

NIH	National Institutes of Health
OA	osteoarthritis
PTSD	post-traumatic stress disorder
RA	rheumatoid arthritis
RANTES	regulated on activation, normal T-cell expressed and secreted
SSA	Social Security Administration
SSRI	selective serotonin reuptake inhibitor
VA	Department of Veterans Affairs
WHO	World Health Organization

1

Introduction[1]

The Social Security Act defines disability as

the inability to engage in any substantial gainful activity by reason of any medically determinable physical or mental impairment(s) which can be expected to result in death or which has lasted or can be expected to last for a continuous period of not less than 12 months. (SSA, 2020)

As part of the overall disability determination process, the Social Security Administration (SSA) uses a step-by-step approach to understand how severe an individual's condition is and whether it meets program criteria for disability. The use of various types of biomarkers has been suggested as a way to strengthen the amount and quality of objective evidence available to the review process.

Recognizing the practical value biomarkers may have in disability adjudication, SSA asked the National Academies of Sciences, Engineering, and Medicine's (the National Academies') Board on Health Care Services to organize a workshop titled The State of the Science of the Use of Biomarkers to Establish the Presence and Severity of Impairments. As

---

[1] The planning committee's role was limited to planning the workshop, and the Proceedings of a Workshop was prepared by the workshop rapporteurs as a factual summary of what occurred at the workshop. Statements, recommendations, and opinions expressed are those of individual presenters and participants and are not necessarily endorsed or verified by the National Academies of Sciences, Engineering, and Medicine, and they should not be construed as reflecting any group consensus.

part of its charge, SSA asked the National Academies to organize general discussions around:

- The current use and potential uses for biomarkers in general;
- The current clinical use of biomarkers by health care professionals to determine function or impairment severity; and
- The legal and ethical implications associated with biomarker use in clinical decision making.

Furthermore, SSA asked the National Academies to focus on the use of non-genetic biomarkers as tools for the diagnosis or prognosis of the severity of six specific physical and mental impairments: fibromyalgia, arthritis, post-traumatic stress disorder (PTSD), major depression, schizophrenia, and chronic pain. The workshop was held virtually on July 21, 2020.

BACKGROUND

In the opening remarks at the workshop, Mark Warshawsky, deputy commissioner for retirement and disability policy at SSA, said, "SSA is always looking for ways to enhance our services to the public." SSA is "committed to incorporating advances in medical sciences and technology" into the body of evidence, he explained, adding, "The use of biomarkers in identification and management of various health conditions is an emerging science with the potential to make a significant impact on the delivery of health care."

In the process of understanding how these biomarkers would fit into the adjudication process, "we first require objective medical evidence to establish a medically determinable impairment," Warshawsky continued. It is also necessary to consider the severity and duration of the impairment, or whether the individual has multiple impairments, he added. For its purposes, he said SSA "would like to know how biomarkers could serve as objective medical evidence to help make accurate, timely, and evidence-based decisions for claimants on a larger scale." Essentially, he noted, SSA wants to know if it is possible to link biomarkers to function, as well as potential ethical and legal implications. He explained that SSA chose the six mental and physical conditions being presented at the workshop "because they appear frequently in applications for disability benefits and can be especially challenging to adjudicate."

ORGANIZATION OF PROCEEDINGS

This proceedings document is organized into five chapters. Following the introduction with background on the charge from SSA, Chapter

2 presents an overview of how biomarkers are used and their potential for the diagnosis and prognosis of health and functionality. Chapter 3 reviews the state of the science for various biomarkers across several specific impairments, and Chapter 4 incorporates perspectives on legal and ethical implications for the use of biomarkers in clinical decision making. Chapter 5 provides final thoughts and suggestions for the use of biomarkers within SSA for disability determination. Appendix A includes the Statement of Task for the workshop. The workshop agenda is provided in Appendix B, and biographical sketches of the workshop speakers and planning committee members are found in Appendix C. Speakers' presentations and the webcast have been archived online.[2]

---

[2] See https://www.nationalacademies.org/event/03-30-2020/the-use-of-biomarkers-to-establish-presence-and-severity-of-impairments-a-workshop (accessed September 3, 2020).

2

Understanding Biomarker Use and Its Potential for Determining Health and Function

Key Messages from Individual Speakers and Participants
- Biomarkers are objectively measured characteristics that are used as an indicator of normal biological processes, the presence of disease, or pharmacologic responses to a therapeutic intervention (Menetski).
- The rigorous process of developing a biomarker can be as resource intensive as drug development and is specific to the type of biomarker being developed (Menetski).
- Using the World Health Organization *International Classification of Functioning, Disability and Health* framework in biomarker usage can improve the precision of care as the framework incorporates personal and environmental factors that can moderate function, and ultimately, quality of life (Wagner).
- More precise biomarker characterizations are needed to further integrate biomarkers into standard clinical practice (Menetski, Wagner).

To understand the potential role of biomarkers in disability determination, it is first necessary to define biomarkers and explore their potential use in the diagnosis and prognosis of health and function in general. In the first panel of the workshop, Joseph Menetski, associate vice president of Research Partnerships at the Foundation for the National Institutes of Health (FNIH), discussed the history and definition of biomarkers broadly. Amy Wagner, professor of neuroscience and Endowed Chair for Translational Research at the University of Pittsburgh, followed by presenting how biomarkers relate to health and function. The panel concluded with a discussion, led by Sara Rosenbaum, Harold and Jane Hirsh professor of Health, Law, and Policy at The George Washington University, on challenges in the development and advancement of biomarkers, as well as the importance of the context of use (COU). This chapter reviews the history and current uses of biomarkers, how they relate to health and function, and their future development and challenges in COU.

HISTORY AND DEFINITION OF BIOMARKERS

Menetski started with an overview of FNIH's work with biomarkers. The goal of FNIH, he stated, is "to attract and share resources and create consensus." This is done through the various public–private partnerships it facilitates, such as the Biomarkers Consortium. The Biomarkers Consortium has raised more than $95 million over the past 12 years to fund partnerships that involve a wide array of public and private stakeholders such as the Food and Drug Administration (FDA), the National Institutes of Health (NIH), the Centers for Medicare & Medicaid Services, the Pharmaceutical Research and Manufacturers of America, other pharmaceutical and nutritional companies, and not-for-profit organizations (Menetski et al., 2019). The consortium was created because of the novelty of the field of biomarkers and the need for regulation, he explained. FNIH efforts, he said, have created and led cross-sector efforts that validate and qualify biomarkers and other drug development tools to accelerate decision making for the development of new therapeutics and health technologies. So far, the Biomarkers Consortium has contributed to the advancement of 14 therapeutics and generated tools being used in drug development (FNIH, 2020; Menetski et al., 2019); these efforts have greatly improved the field of biomarkers.

Biomarkers Overview

Menetski continued by discussing the definition and classification of biomarkers. He found that the definitions of key terms in biomarker research provided by SSA are similar to the definitions included in the Biomarkers, EndpointS and other Tools (BEST) glossary, which was created by FDA and NIH (see Box 2-1).

Biomarker Classification

Biomarkers can be classified into seven categories (FDA-NIH Biomarker Working Group, 2016), said Menetski. The first three categories—susceptibility and risk biomarkers, diagnostic biomarkers, and prognostic biomarkers—are used to measure disease presence and status. The additional four categories—monitoring biomarkers, predictive biomarkers, pharmacodynamic and response biomarkers, and safety biomarkers—are used to measure aspects of response to treatment. He offered various examples of biomarkers and their classifications (see Table 2-1).

BOX 2-1
Definitions of Key Terms in Biomarker Research

Select terms and definitions provided by the Social Security Administration for verification include:

- Biomarker: A characteristic that is objectively measured and evaluated as an indicator of normal biological processes, the presence of disease, or pharmacologic responses to a therapeutic intervention.
- Clinical endpoint: A variable that characterizes a study subject's well-being from his or her perspective (i.e., how the subject thinks he or she feels or functions).

Select terms and definitions from the Biomarkers, EndpointS, and other Tools (BEST) glossary (FDA-NIH Biomarker Working Group, 2016) are:

- A biomarker is "a characteristic that is measured as an indicator of normal biological processes, pathogenic processes, or biological responses to an exposure or intervention, including therapeutic interventions." These can be molecular, histologic, radiographic, or physiologic characteristics.
- A clinical endpoint is "a precisely defined variable intended to reflect an outcome of interest that is statistically analyzed to address a particular research question."
- A clinical outcome is "an outcome that describes or reflects how an individual feels, functions, or survives."
- A clinical outcome assessment (COA) is an "assessment of a clinical outcome [that] can be made through report by a clinician, a patient, a nonclinician observer, or a performance-based assessment. There are four types of COAs: clinician-reported outcome, observer-reported outcome, patient-reported outcome, and performance outcome."

SOURCE: Joseph Menetski presentation, July 21, 2020.

TABLE 2-1 Examples of Biomarkers and Their Key Uses

Biomarkers	Examples	Key Uses
Susceptibility and risk biomarkers	• Body mass index or 2-hour postmeal glucose for diabetes risk • Apolipoprotein E genotype risk for Alzheimer's disease	• Define population for more efficient prevention trials
Diagnostic biomarkers	• Blood pressure in hypertension • Forced expiratory volume for chronic obstructive pulmonary disease	• Define disease population for study
Prognostic biomarkers	• Gleason score in prostate cancer • Total kidney volume in autosomal dominant polycystic kidney disease	• Define higher-risk disease population, enhancing trial efficiency
Monitoring biomarkers	• Hepatitis C virus-ribonucleic acid • Prostate-specific antigen in prostate cancer	• Monitor patient status in trials
Predictive biomarkers	• Cystic fibrosis genotypes response to ivacaftor • Microsatellite-high predicts response to pembrolizumab	• Trial enrichment improves efficiency, reduces sample size, and increases response to treatment
Pharmacodynamic and response biomarkers	• Blood pressure in hypertension • Forced expiratory volume or 6-minute walk test • Low density lipoprotein cholesterol	• Demonstrating drug-target engagement and dose-ranging • Surrogate endpoints (validated or reasonably likely)
Safety biomarkers	• Alanine aminotransferase, creatinine, estimated glomerular filtration rate • Urinary kidney injury biomarkers (e.g., KIM-1)	• Detecting and assessing drug toxicity

NOTE: KIM-1 = kidney injury molecule 1.
SOURCES: Joseph Menetski presentation, July 21, 2020. Adapted from Stein, 2020. Information from FDA-NIH Biomarker Working Group, 2016.

Evidentiary Criteria Framework

Building on the examples, Menetski described the evidentiary criteria framework, which is used to determine biomarker qualification (if enough data are present to use a biomarker) and provide a consistent set of characteristics to describe and define the biomarker program with a regulatory agency, such as FDA (Leptak et al., 2017). The goal of the framework is to enhance submission quality and predictability of the qualification process, and clarify the type and amount of evidentiary criteria needed. Menetski described the framework as a five-component process:

1. Identifying the need statement (i.e., what is the knowledge gap?);
2. Defining the COU (i.e., what question is the biomarker addressing, what information will it provide, and/or what is the specific fit-for-purpose use?);
3. Determining the benefit (e.g., improved sensitivity);
4. Determining the risk (e.g., consequences of false positives or false negatives); and
5. Defining the evidentiary criteria, using analytical and clinical validation:
    a. Analytical validation is used to determine whether the performance characteristics of the biomarker test are acceptable for the proposed COU.
    b. Clinical validation is used to determine whether the correlation between the biomarker and the outcome of interest are acceptable for the proposed COU (CDER, 2018; Leptak et al., 2017).

Biomarker Development in the Drug Development Process

To conclude, Menetski acknowledged that biomarker development can be as difficult and as resource intensive as drug development. He noted that the correlation of a biomarker to a clinical observation is only as good as the precision that the observation can be quantified, and he emphasized that the type of biomarker being developed will dictate the type of data that are needed to ensure confident decision making. He stated that a biomarker is not the tool used to measure it. For example, "Blood pressure is a biomarker. It does not matter how you measure blood pressure," Menetski said. "The biomarker is the actual analyte, or the actual measurement. It is not how you make the measurement," he concluded, so there may be various methods to detect a given biomarker.

RELATING BIOMARKERS TO HEALTH AND FUNCTION

Wagner began by defining health and function as concepts and then discussed the World Health Organization's (WHO's) *International Classification of Functioning, Disability and Health* (ICF) framework to demonstrate how biomarkers can be used as tools in research (see Figure 2-1). She then highlighted ways to move forward in biomarker research and initiatives and programs that use biomarkers for functional assessment.

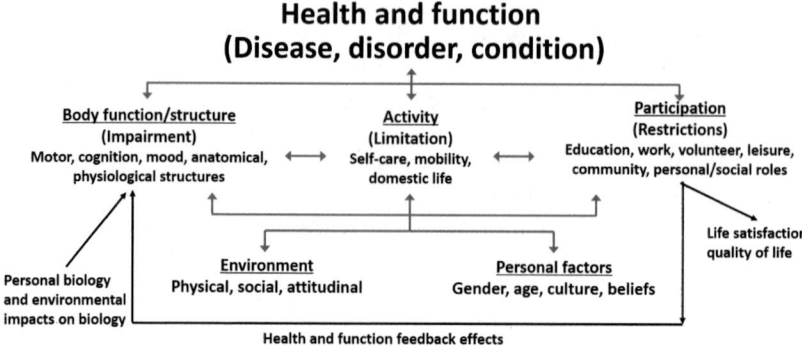

FIGURE 2-1 The World Health Organization's *International Classification of Functioning, Disability and Health* model.
SOURCES: Amy Wagner presentation, July 21, 2020. Adapted from WHO, 2002.

Health and Function Conceptualized

Wagner offered three definitions of health from Sartorius (2006), beginning with the absence of disease, which she stated "is most relevant to the medical model and is based on the state of science, signs, and symptoms." She acknowledged that this is likely the most widely accepted definition of health in the health care field. The second definition describes health as "a state that allows individuals to adequately cope with all demands of life." She added, "This definition is important because it begins to make assumptions about health that are based on level of function."

The third definition of health is "a state of balance or equilibrium between individuals and their social and physical environments." She emphasized the importance of this third definition because "here, health reflects an internal equilibrium to get the most from life despite disease, and inherent to this definition then is the incorporation of values that individuals have about their cultures and communities." Based on these definitions, Wagner concluded that health and function are interrelated, and multiple elements should be considered in terms of functioning. Biomarker research occurs within this complex landscape.

The WHO International Classification of Functioning, Disability and Health *Framework*

Wagner continued by elaborating on WHO's ICF, which provides a standard language and framework for measuring and categorizing functioning and disability, in the context of health (WHO, 2001). It is focused on impairments, activities, and participation. Impairments are defined as problems with body functions and structures that are associated with health conditions. Types of impairments include emotional, motor, cognitive, or other sensory functions. Wagner pointed out that these impairments can "lead to symptoms such as cognitive dysfunction, balance deficits, paralysis, and changes in mood that can be related to common diseases associated with disability assessments, such as dementia, post-traumatic stress disorder, stroke, schizophrenia, spinal cord injury, traumatic brain injury, and degenerative joint disease." From this first element of the WHO ICF, Wagner said, we can "link symptoms to disease."

The second element of the WHO ICF is characterized by activities, which are "things individuals do to be independent members of the community," she said. She said that activities are

> focused on execution of a daily task or action and are things we need to do to care for ourselves and carry out our goals in life. This includes various aspects such as functional mobility, household management, recreation, work, personal care, and learning new skills. These activities help us fulfill our wants and needs.

The third defining element of the WHO ICF is participation. This element "is distinguished from activity through the ideas of intent and impact," said Wagner, adding that "participation focuses more on involvement in a life situation and is related to the various roles we assume in our daily lives." Participation encompasses meaningful engagement, personal and societal responsibility, making an impact on others, taking advantage of access and opportunities, and social connectedness and inclusion. These factors highlight "the idea of respect and dignity resulting from participating fully in all areas of our lives," she said. She offered the everyday scenario of getting dressed as an example to differentiate activities and participation. One might define "getting dressed as an activity, but getting dressed to go to the prom or a job interview is participation because you are engaging with others in social connectedness and social roles," she explained.

Wagner said the ICF framework also incorporates the idea that both personal factors and environmental factors can moderate daily functions across multiple dimensions. She further emphasized that functioning at the fullest level affects life satisfaction and quality of life.

Tools for Measuring Health and Function

Wagner explained how the WHO ICF framework can be used to link biomarkers to function by using it to help understand how biomarkers relate to rehabilitation processes. She explained further:

The framework has allowed novel opportunities to work toward precision care for populations with disabilities in terms of diagnostic and prognostic markers, biomarker-guided clinical decision algorithms, and biosusceptibility tools for screening prevention, as well as biological stratification for clinical trials.

Milleville et al. (2019) found that inflammation in a population with traumatic brain injury contributed substantially to cognitive dysfunction. Downstream effects from the inflammatory burden were also noted and helped researchers understand more about its impact on daily functions that require cognitive capacity, as well as its indirect impact on quality of life. This work was provided as an example of the role biomarkers can play in "bridging the gap between health and function," said Wagner.

Envisioning a Future Path and Leveraging Existing Resources

Wagner discussed the long-term goal for biomarker use of helping people monitor and manage their health and function. One way this may happen is through the use of point-of-care technologies and telehealth tools where information can be entered into a large data infrastructure that would provide personalized readouts for the individuals needing care. She acknowledged the immense progress needed to reach this goal, but she also highlighted existing resources that will help bridge the gap, such as the Precision Medicine Initiative, All of Us Research Program, and the Million Veteran Program (MVP).

Wagner reviewed the NIH Precision Medicine Initiative that was launched in 2015 by President Obama;[1] she explained that it is a long-time research endeavor whose goal is to improve understanding of individualized approaches to disease and treatment. The initiative's short-term focus is cancer, and its long-term focus is intended to encompass all areas of health and disease (Collins and Varmus, 2015). Wagner believes potential opportunities exist to "use this type of resource to learn more about how disability and functioning can be prioritized as a focus of biomarkers research."

Wagner elaborated on the All of Us Research Program,[2] a program within the Precision Medicine Initiative. The goal of this program is to improve and personalize the ways health conditions are prevented, diagnosed, and treated (All of Us Research Program Investigators, 2019). The program intends to build a database of 1 million individuals with

---

[1] See https://ghr.nlm.nih.gov/primer/precisionmedicine/initiative (accessed September 8, 2020).

[2] See https://allofus.nih.gov (accessed September 8, 2020).

genomic biomarker and health care information to study various areas where personal biology can inform clinical care. "The program focuses on genomic heterogeneity and personal biology to better understand disease mechanisms," said Wagner. The National Center for Medical Rehabilitation Research has also been involved with the All of Us Research Program "by incorporating principles of health and function within enrollment processes and research efforts," she said. Further opportunities exist for "large-scale studies to address biomarkers as functional assessment tools," but she pointed out that it will require ongoing engagement with disability researchers and consumers on barriers to participation, as well as continued engagement with disability advocates and populations to prioritize focus within the research.

The final resource Wagner highlighted is the Department of Veterans Affairs' (VA's) MVP,[3] which launched in 2011. The goal of the MVP is to "learn more about how genes, lifestyle, and military exposures particularly affect health and function" (VA, 2020). The program has enrolled 825,000 individuals (VA, 2020) and partnered with other entities such as the Department of Energy for its Big Data Science Initiative. The MVP has "created a large biobank for future use in various areas of research [available to VA researchers]," said Wagner, and it has "a variety of ongoing research programs that center on the idea of individualized approaches to disease diagnosis and management." She noted that significant opportunities exist for consumer engagement in defining and assessing the genomics that might be affecting function.

DISCUSSION

Rosenbaum moderated a discussion on challenges in the development of biomarkers and important future considerations. Workshop participants and planning committee members posed questions related to progress in biomarkers research and discussed various factors that should be considered when implementing biomarkers in practice.

Challenges in Development and Advancement of Biomarkers

Rosenbaum asked the panelists about the timeline of implementing biomarker research into standard practice. "There is still a lot to be done in terms of characterizing biomarker relationships to disease and drug development," Wagner replied. She emphasized the need to strengthen these characterizations to be able to map them onto disease-specific func-

---

[3] See https://www.mvp.va.gov/webapp/mvp-web-participant/#/public (accessed September 8, 2020).

tions. Menetski supported Wagner and said, "Many existing definitions of disease are not precise enough to address," and there is a "need to look at the process of redefining diseases so a strong comparative baseline exists from which to make quantitative measures."

Srinivasa Murthy, a retired psychiatry professor, posed a question on the development of pain as a biomarker. Wagner explained that the challenge of using pain as a biomarker, versus factors such as oxygen or cholesterol, is that pain is a self-reported, subjective phenomenon. She noted

> There is still much to be learned about the substrates of pain and the complexities that go into translating a biomarker to a self-reported subjective measure, but areas such as neuroimaging have been useful in bridging the gap.

Menetski added that "pain as a biomarker relates to precision in measuring." For example, he explained, people with arthritis often categorize various pains (e.g., back pain, knee pain) in the same way, even though pain can vary.

Robert Wallace, emeritus professor of epidemiology and internal medicine at the University of Iowa, enquired about the regulatory pathway to deep learning-based biomarker discovery. In response, Menetski acknowledged the investments that have been made in artificial intelligence by looking at multianalytes, such as omic technology. FDA requires a more comprehensive understanding of the process of using omic technology to produce a reliable biomarker score. Multiple variables are involved in calculating each biomarker score, which can complicate regulation, Menetski said.

Importance of Context of Use

Questions were posed by workshop participants regarding parameters that exist between people who exhibit biomarkers and those who do not, as well as biomarkers that are not readily tied to pathophysiology but have a strong association with a clinical outcome measure. Menetski responded by emphasizing the importance of COU in both scenarios. He explained that biomarkers can require varying levels of precision and that accuracy also factors into each scenario, as explained in the evidentiary criteria framework. Using cholesterol as an example, he explained that a biomarker could have long-term effects and require less precision in measuring versus oxygen levels that could have more immediate effects.

Continuing the topic of COU, workshop participants asked about the role of demographic factors such as age, environment, race, and ethnicity in biomarker use and validation. Wagner noted that the interplay between age and environment is complex because "as our bodies age, we have more environmental exposures." Because of this, "there is not going to be a one-size-fits-all approach in how biomarkers are applied based on age, gender, or similar factors," and that these factors are taken into consideration in biomarker development, she said. Wagner and Menetski both agreed that race and ethnicity play a role as well. Wagner said, "There are some biological differences that come in part as a result of our personal biology that we inherit over the generations, and race and ethnic background can factor into that." Other factors, such as access to health care and health care maintenance and prevention, also play a role in understanding and applying biomarkers, said Wagner. Together, these all create a complex environment that we will need to navigate when using these biomarkers to try and understand disease and function more clearly, she added.

3

State of the Science for Specific Impairments

Key Messages from Individual Speakers and Participants

- For most multifactorial diseases and syndromes, there will be no single biomarker to rely on for diagnosis, prognosis, treatment, etc. (Sowa).
- Future directions should include prospective trials to validate tools and align biomarker expectations with the Food and Drug Administration (Etkin, Lieberman, Trivedi).
- Cognitive assessment could be a cost-effective predictor of disability in schizophrenia (Harvey).
- There is no chronic pain condition where there is a good relationship between anything peripherally measurable (e.g., radiograph or magnetic resonance imaging) and the presence or severity of pain, primarily because pain occurs from a number of biopsychosocial factors not typically assessed or treated in clinical practice (Clauw).
- Emphasis on biomarkers (such as radiological biomarkers), instead of the patient's pain and activity levels, can lead to overmedication and overtreatment (Bathon, Sowa).
- The pathogenesis of osteoarthritis is complex and multifactorial, yet trials are often focused on a single joint with standardized imaging and pain reporting (Kraus).
- The utility of a biomarker may depend on the stage and natural history of the disease (Bathon, Kraus, Sowa).

Several impairments that are commonly cited in applications for disability are challenging to assess. With these impairments in mind, SSA requested updates on the state of the science for the potential use of biomarkers to assist in the determination process. Speakers presented research and clinical insight on major depression, PTSD, schizophrenia, fibromyalgia, rheumatoid arthritis (RA), osteoarthritis (OA), and back pain. This chapter reviews their presentations and the ensuing discussions.

MAJOR DEPRESSION

Madhukar Trivedi, founding director for the Center for Depression Research and Clinical Care at the University of Texas Southwestern Medical Center at Dallas, explained that the issue with biomarkers is two-fold. He said, "We need to have a better sense of the accuracy of the biomarker used," and "what is the replicability of the biomarker, so that it can be used in scalable forms." He presented his work on major depression, saying it is a chronic and heterogeneous disorder, and researchers are beginning to make progress on biomarkers for diagnosis and severity of disease, but "it is still a little early" to rely on biomarkers for diagnosis of depression. However, treatment-matching biomarkers are closer for widespread use, he said. The most promising biomarkers in depression are inflammatory biomarkers (e.g., C-reactive protein, IL1-beta, gene expression) and neuroimaging biomarkers (functional magnetic resonance imaging [fMRI], electroencephalogram [EEG]), but he noted that there is increasing evidence coming from metabolic markers and the gut microbiome to help with treatment metrics.

Inflammatory Biomarkers

Trivedi said, "There is now very strong evidence that a proportion of patients with depression, probably between 20 and 30 percent, have some evidence of low-level inflammation that can be identified," with consistency across several studies (Osimo et al., 2020). Trivedi also referenced a meta-analysis review on reward processing in depressed patients compared to healthy controls, which found consistent neural aberrations in imaging in the depressed patients (Keren et al., 2018). He cautioned that "there have been significant false starts in the field when examining biomarkers for depression, primarily because most of the studies were looking at biomarkers after the studies were completed." There are also few studies that look at biomarkers to differentiate outcomes between drug and placebo interventions. A challenge with understanding biomarkers for depression is that most studies look at a single treatment, which can give some idea of prognostic indicators, but the lack of comparison groups makes it difficult for clinicians to identify the best treatment, he said. From his perspective:

> The best biomarkers for treatment matching are those that can tell you to select treatment A and avoid treatment B. This is what is really needed in order to be used in clinical practice.

One biomarker that Trivedi thought is worthwhile for treatment selection is C-reactive protein. For example, the Combining Medications to Enhance Depression Outcomes (CO-MED) trial compared outcomes for patients who were given either a selective serotonin reuptake inhibitor (SSRI) monotherapy, or bupropion plus the SSRI monotherapy. The study found that in patients where C-reactive protein is not disturbed (< 1 mg/L), the SSRI is the more effective treatment, but if C-reactive protein is equal to or more than 1 mg/L, the bupropion-SSRI combination is the more effective treatment (Jha et al., 2017). Trivedi argued that C-reactive protein is an important biomarker to consider, as without it, "we are blindly selecting patients for treatment, which is just a trial and error process."

As another example of using an inflammatory marker for intervention, he shared a study exploring aerobic exercise as a treatment augmentation for patients with major depressive disorder who did not respond to SSRIs (Trivedi et al., 2011). In the study, the higher-dose exercise group showed a trend of higher remission rates compared to a group with a lower dose of exercise. But, upon further examination, the researchers found that only those patients with elevated levels of TNF-alpha actually had the best improvement with exercise (Trivedi et al., 2011). In other words, Trivedi said, "The anti-inflammatory effects of exercise may be effective for [treating] depression, but only if there is some elevation in inflammation, as measured in this study, at least through TNF-alpha."

Brain-Based Biomarkers

Trivedi shared a recently published EEG study he worked on with Amit Etkin, chief executive officer at Alto Neuroscience, which used a machine-learning approach to predict antidepressant response in major depression (Wu et al., 2020). Previously, EEG machine-learning studies had challenges related to volume conduction, reduced dimensionality, and signal optimization, said Trivedi (Wu et al., 2020). However, Wu et al. (2020) were able to develop a machine-learning algorithm to address these three problems. When applied to data from an imaging-coupled, placebo-controlled antidepressant study, the algorithm predicted symptom improvement for those patients on sertraline and predicted no improvement for those on placebo (Wu et al., 2020). The algorithm was also generalizable across study sites and equipment. These findings suggest a clinical avenue for a more tailored and personalized treatment for depression, said Trivedi.

Etkin elaborated on this study by asking, when thinking about EEG as a biomarker, how do you take this information and merge it with biology to produce some type of meaningful answer that has valuable clinical implications? A large part of the answer will be machine learning (a form of artificial intelligence), he said. Specifically, he described two approaches: supervised and unsupervised. In a supervised approach, "you take data and put it through a specific algorithm to predict a known outcome and [it] tries to understand the heterogeneity in outcomes," said Etkin. Conversely, he said, an unsupervised approach "is much more discovery oriented, and takes the same data but uses a different type of algorithm that tries to understand the heterogeneity of the biology itself, and then relates that to the outcome." To answer his original question, Etkin shared that when you split the participants by EEG signature, the results within quartiles of response rate for sertraline when compared to the response rate for the placebo are much different than when they are all grouped together and compared to placebo (Fonzo et al., 2019; Wu et al., 2020) (see Figure 3-1).

Etkin said EEG machine learning can help identify people who would be responsive to a particular intervention. Typically, he said,

> people who would come into a clinic for treatment might have very similar symptoms, but only a minority of them would respond to treatment. Therefore, that minority might drive a drug trial to show positive or negative results.

But when the group is disaggregated, the responses to a given treatment may be much larger. Additionally, Etkin said that these "various EEG signatures have no relation to depression severity at baseline." The brain is able to make predictions that do not relate to how the disorder is characterized clinically at baseline, he elaborated.

In summary, Trivedi said that no single biomarker is likely to account for a larger population of patients with depression. Instead, it is likely that a combination of biomarkers will be needed for the best understanding. While most depressed patients do not achieve remission with the first prescribed antidepressant, "that does not mean that the second, third, or fourth treatment will not work," he noted. Instead of the trial-and-error process used currently, using biomarkers to match patients to treatment

STATE OF THE SCIENCE FOR SPECIFIC IMPAIRMENTS

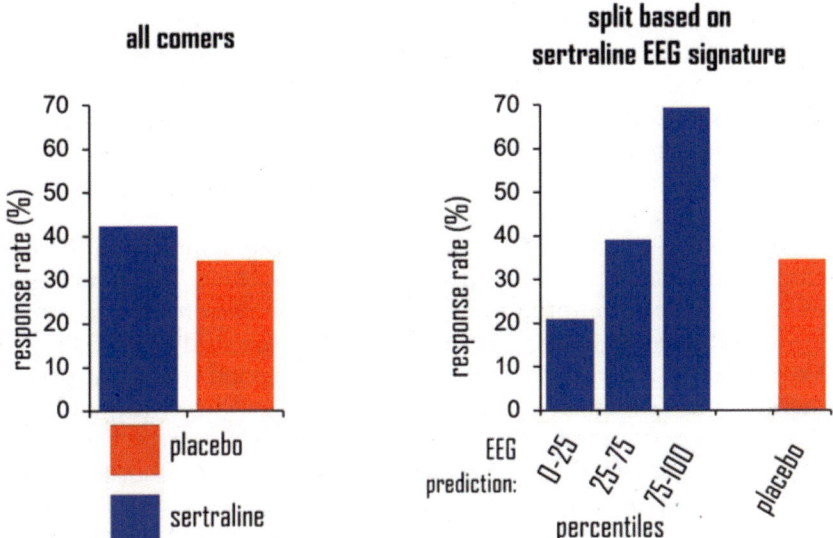

FIGURE 3-1 Supervised prediction of treatment outcome.
NOTE: EEG = electroencephalogram.
SOURCES: Amit Etkin presentation, July 21, 2020. Data from Fonzo et al., 2019; Wu et al., 2020.

can be a way to help patients achieve remission much faster. Etkin suggested that "You can train a machine-learning classifier to detect a certain subtype in one cohort and apply it to another with 90 percent accuracy, consistently." He added that replicability and robustness are important guiding factors for biomarker development and use. Trivedi said the field cannot "just depend on prognostic or predictive biomarkers," but really needs to "look for moderators to help differentiate treatments" in order to advance. In the future, Trivedi said, this work can be used in prevention or at early onset of treatment, ideally leading to better outcomes.

POST-TRAUMATIC STRESS DISORDER

Etkin elaborated on network connectivity, describing a study by Zhang et al. (2020) that characterized individuals with depression or with PTSD using an unsupervised clustering approach to examine only their EEG data to try and understand the heterogeneity between patients. He said the study found a difference in connectivity patterns between healthy participants and those with a disease, but more notably, upon closer examination, there are consistently two clusters of patients that are quite different.

The first cluster looks fairly similar to healthy participants, he explained, but the second cluster looks completely different. Zhang et al. (2020) were able to identify these two clusters in the four different cohorts that were examined, representing two different diseases—depression and PTSD. Etkin said the connectivity differences between the two clusters are heavily focused in the frontal and parietal cortex, regions in the brain important for cognitive control and attention. But all four cohorts look similar to one another, he noted.

In the PTSD sample, the study included a population of individuals entering psychotherapy-based treatment at a VA clinic. This intervention uses a biological approach by working with the person's brain circuitry through the course of therapy. Etkin said that the study found that just like sertraline, individuals who are subtype 1 respond well to the psychotherapy intervention, but those in subtype 2 do not really respond at all. Interestingly, he added, this is independent of therapy type because the study included two different types of therapies in the cohorts and both had the same results.

In summary, Etkin said that by taking an assessment tool (e.g., EEG) used in the clinic and systematically organizing the machine learning and development of signals, it is possible to create a series of brain signatures that can accurately inform clinical decisions in different ways. But these decisions are distinct from clinical measures, as he pointed out that these findings did not relate to baseline severity of symptoms or relate to subtyping based on clinical rounds. There is something uniquely important in the biology, he said, that cuts through the clinical heterogeneity, which has been challenging in the past. He saw the near-term applicability of this approach as exciting for treatment selection and long-term prognosis.

SCHIZOPHRENIA

"Mental disorders are one of the only areas in medicine that do not have the majority of conditions diagnostically confirmed by pathological measure of illness," declared Jeffrey Lieberman, professor and chairman of psychiatry at Columbia University. The only two exceptions are Alzheimer's disease and narcolepsy, he added. One of the first biomarkers associated with mental disorders was identified in 1967, when cerebral plaque findings in deceased patients were correlated with dementia severity and cognition (Roth et al., 1967). This study informed the field and set the stage for further growth, especially in the area of dementias, he said. "Hopefully, other mental illnesses will be able to learn more from biomarkers," he added.

"Schizophrenia is a particularly tragic disease because it begins when people are coming into the prime of their lives," Lieberman said. "If they are not able to find effective treatment, they can experience deterioration in intellectual function, leading to a chronic end stage of illness where they become functionally impaired. So, the goal is to successfully identify people as early as possible and intervene to prevent this progression," he explained. "Biomarkers would be very valuable in this process," he said, and he described three main themes that emerge from 100 years of research on schizophrenia. First, "Schizophrenia runs in families and so is presumed to be genetic." Second, it involves neurochemical transmission—more specifically the neurotransmitters dopamine, glutamate, and gamma aminobutyric acid (GABA) are most prominently implicated. Finally, he said

> It affects brain structure, but it does not devastate the brain diffusely. The main areas implicated through a variety of research are the midbrain—where dopamine neurons are located, the frontal cortex—associated with higher mental functions, and the hippocampus, which is critical in several ways.

Dopamine dysregulation in presynaptic trafficking and release has been conclusively demonstrated in schizophrenic patients (Laruelle et al., 2003; Sulzer et al., 2000), Lieberman said. "But its utility as a biomarker is limited because the dysregulation is only seen during acute phases of the illness and does not always distinguish people with schizophrenia from healthy controls," he noted. Additionally, using positron emission tomography (PET) scans to detect this dysregulation is expensive and cumbersome, he added. Cassidy et al. (2019) identified neuromelanin as a potential indicator because deposition of neuromelanin in the midbrain area is also seen as a measure of excessive dopamine, said Lieberman. Neuromelanin can be detected using simpler imaging, and its presence in the mid-brain as a biomarker of dopamine has been validated in postmortem brains. Sulzer et al. (2000) also found neuromelanin to be associated with the severity of schizophrenia symptoms. Lieberman noted that the study researchers suggest that neuromelanin can be useful as a diagnostic measure and potentially as a prognostic measure as well.

Hippocampal Biomarkers

"The hippocampus is one of the earliest structures in the brain to be affected by schizophrenia," said Lieberman, "but it is a very complex area." Based on prior research, Lieberman and his colleagues have been able to focus on the CA1 subregion of the hippocampus for biomarker efforts. The model is based on glutamate because there is potential excess release of glutamate that leads to a chain reaction resulting in potential cell atrophy. Deterioration associated with schizophrenia begins here, he explained. From a biomarker standpoint, he said there are imaging modalities that can be used to detect this deterioration, but brain changes detected by imaging often come too late in the disease progression to have strong mitigation opportunities. Another method that is promising is using spectroscopy, Lieberman said, which involves comparing GABA peaks on spectroscopic resonance imaging between clinically high-risk patients who do not have the illness yet and healthy controls. Research shows that the measure of metabolic activity of the cells in the CA1 region of the hippocampus is elevated in patients in all aspects compared to controls, but there is no difference in volume, meaning that the disease has not yet progressed to the point of structural pathology changes.

If these high-risk patients are followed, Lieberman said, "We find that the progression is not associated with the combined signal of glutamine and glutamate, but it is associated with GABA." The correlation with symptoms is also very high with GABA. Lieberman said he believes that the profile of these measures can be validated as predictive, but what is most predictive of severe disease is the atrophy of the brain volume. Those patients with the most loss of volume have the highest rate of progression to syndromal psychosis, he added.

Biomarkers for Functional Capacity and Disability

Philip Harvey, professor of psychiatry at the University of Miami, centered his presentation on biomarkers that he said are easily detectable, readily measurable, and have strong prognostic implications. Harvey et al. (2012) looked at people who were immediately approved for disability compensation compared to those whose claims were adjudicated and subsequently either reconsidered or dropped. What the study found, he explained, is that the majority of those who are approved receive compensation immediately, but a significant number of individuals undergo a lengthy and expensive adjudication process, even though they are awarded compensation in the end (Harvey et al., 2012). Many unsuccessful initial applicants are not denied, he said, but are unable to complete the process and would likely benefit from a more objective marker. Cognitive impairment in schizophrenia is quite substantial, Harvey noted, with the average level representing an IQ score of 63. But the challenge is that many psychiatric professionals do not routinely perform cognitive assessments. For example, Keefe et al. (2006) measured correlation between performance-based cognition and functional capacity based on interviews with caregivers or people close to the patients. The study shows that subjective assessment of disability is important, but it does not correlate with objective information, he said.

"Cognition is clearly a biomarker," he said, and because "impairment is fully developed by the time the first psychotic symptoms are identified it can be useful as an early predictive indicator of risk for disability compensation." Harvey noted that those with considerable cognitive symptoms at their first episode of schizophrenia have only about a 14 percent chance of functional recovery 5 years later (Robinson et al., 2004), and those symptoms should be considered a first line biomarker for prediction of SSA disability status.

Beyond cognition, Harvey added that negative symptoms in schizophrenia are also important to consider and come in several forms. These include reduced emotional experience, which is highly related to social drive and functioning; blunted affect; reduced volume of speech; and reduced intonation (Ventura et al., 2015, 2019). These symptoms are often highly visible to observers, he said, and are an early marker of risk for schizophrenia. For example, studies suggest that negative symptoms at the time of a first psychotic episode can predict 8-year functional outcomes (Ventura et al., 2015, 2019), with similar predictive power as cognition. But this assessment of negative symptoms is challenging and requires clinical experience, he said, so simply asking family members may not be enough.

He shared some emerging strategies focused on "digital biomarkers" for negative symptoms in schizophrenia, and highlighted paging strategies. This approach involves asking people where they are, who they are with, what they are doing, and how they are feeling. He said that because "classic schizophrenia often includes someone who is socially isolated and sitting at home, this kind of assessment can easily detect that." In three studies, the predominant location of people with schizophrenia was at home (Depp et al., 2019; Granholm et al., 2020; Raugh et al., 2020). Using passive measurement strategies—in this case, global positioning system (GPS) indicators of where the patient is located—Depp et al. (2019) found a high correlation between self-reported location and GPS validation. Harvey said these studies validate self-reported studies and support that the use of GPS indicators can serve as a digital biomarker of negative symptoms in schizophrenia.

Another concern with schizophrenia, especially within the context of being at home, socially isolated and inactive, is the development of early onset comorbid conditions such as metabolic syndrome, Harvey continued. Using data collected from the Suffolk County Mental Health Project, Strassnig et al. (2017b) found that patients who were overweight at the onset of their illness were about 60 percent more likely to be obese two decades later. Additionally, Strassnig et al. (2017a) found that body mass index at illness onset predicted employment significantly at the 20-year follow-up, demonstrating the cascade of becoming overweight, then obese, and then having physical limitations that directly interfere with being able to work.

In summary, Harvey stated that cognition, weight, and activity are biological factors that can predict unemployment. These factors can also "be easily measured, present early in the illness, and are directly relevant to work outcomes and labor force participation," he said. He suggested "using this basic approach, paired with clinical indicators, to have a broad way to address biomarkers of disability and schizophrenia."

CHRONIC PAIN AND FIBROMYALGIA

Daniel Clauw, director of the Chronic Pain and Fatigue Research Center at the University of Michigan, said "There is no chronic pain condition where there is a good relationship between anything peripherally measurable (e.g., radiograph or MRI) and the presence or severity of pain." Primarily, he said

> This is because pain occurs from a number of biopsychosocial factors not typically assessed or treated in clinical practice—especially central nervous system (CNS) factors that play a prominent role with disability or chronic pain.

While there are fairly good biomarkers that can measure these specific CNS factors, Clauw questioned whether these factors should be measured at all.

"Fibromyalgia is a condition that has suffered from credibility," he explained, adding that over the past three decades researchers have learned much more about these types of centralized pain conditions. Previously, fibromyalgia was perceived "as a discrete illness characterized by focal areas of tenderness; now, it has really become the poster child for a third new mechanism of pain" called centralized or nociplastic pain, said Clauw. This mechanism also includes other pain conditions like irritable bowel syndrome, temporal mandibular joint disorder, tension headaches, and many others. "They all have prominent pain, but there is generally nothing wrong in the area of the body where the pain is felt," he said. There is now increasing recognition that many common chronic pain conditions are overlapping, with people being subject to multiple types of pain (Maixner et al., 2016). Essentially, Clauw said, "People are developing pain in new areas and getting new diagnostic labels, but they have not developed a fundamentally new problem. Instead, the pain seems to be driven by CNS problems."

Patient-reported outcomes can help with the assessment and diagnosis of fibromyalgia, he said. In many cases, the disability stems beyond pain and encompasses other factors like fatigue, memory, sleep problems, mood problems, and obesity. These collective factors, rather than analyses of the brain, can more likely predict who is disabled by chronic pain. Clauw described two studies that measured whether fibromyalgia is predictive of surgery outcomes and opioid nonresponsiveness in patients. While surgical procedures seek to ameliorate pain by reducing the nociceptive input at the periphery, surgery does not address the pain that comes from the brain. The studies found that for each 1-point increase in a fibromyalgia score, patients were less responsive to both surgery and opioids.

Brummett et al. (2015) found that among patients undergoing knee or hip surgery, each reported a 1-point increase in their fibromyalgia score that was associated with an 18 percent increase in odds of failure to improve by at least 50 percent. Similarly, Janda et al. (2015) found that among women undergoing a hysterectomy, each reported a 1-point increase in their fibromyalgia score that was associated with 7 mg increase in consumption of oral morphine. Clauw said that even after patients with diagnosed fibromyalgia had surgery, the fibromyalgia score remained a powerful predictor, suggesting that the pain is coming more from the CNS than the actual surgical site.

Other techniques, including imaging, can help researchers understand why opioids are not effective for fibromyalgia or other centralized pain states. Clauw shared that using machine learning, López-Solà et al. (2017) found functional imaging (with greater than 90 percent sensitivity and specificity) could differentiate between a patient with fibromyalgia and a healthy control. These machine-learning techniques are promising in identifying subsets of pain patients who may respond differently to different therapies, but these techniques would not be as useful in adjudicating disability. He said, in conclusion, that one of the main problems in the field of chronic pain is that there are two aspects of pain. The first is what causes the pain (e.g., peripheral problem versus CNS problem). The second aspect comes from the fact that "as patients experience the pain for a longer time, they can develop downstream consequences of pain, and these functional consequences can lead to disability and functional impairments," he said.

Over the course of his career, Clauw estimated he has seen thousands of chronic pain patients and has found it far more likely that "patients consider disability because they have received inadequate treatment for their pain, not that they have failed to respond to proper treatment." A confluence of social, environmental, and economic factors plays a bigger role in the exacerbation of chronic pain than just biological factors, he added. "We go to great efforts to identify the people who are faking their pain," Clauw said, "but in my experience, I can count on one hand the people I have seen like that." Clauw said, "fibromyalgia patients are some of the most disabled people I have seen in rheumatology," but noted that simply putting them on permanent disability may not be the right approach.

He suggested rethinking assessing disability in people with chronic pain by learning from other groups and using care models. For example, the VA uses a care model to identify people with chronic pain in primary care and to aggressively treat them with nonpharmacological therapies. These include manual therapies (e.g., massage, acupuncture), behavioral and psychological therapies (e.g., cognitive behavioral therapy), and exercise and movement therapies (e.g., aerobic exercise, yoga).

ARTHRITIS

Two speakers discussed biomarkers for different types of arthritis. Joan Bathon, chief of the Division of Rheumatology at Columbia University, discussed RA and the current state of biomarkers. Virginia Byers Kraus, professor of medicine, orthopedics, and pathology at the Duke Molecular Physiology Institute, highlighted the challenges with OA.

Rheumatoid Arthritis

Building on Clauw's categorization of pain, Bathon said that RA is more of a nociceptive pain, as it is characterized by joint inflammation, but it can also overlap with fibromyalgia pain. Current biomarkers for RA are limited, but as a general rule, she explained that laboratory biomarkers are not independently adequate for diagnosis, prognosis, or response to treatment for RA. Bathon explained that there is a genetic predisposition to RA. However, she said, the development of RA is a slowly evolving process where patients develop antibodies and an increased level of inflammatory cytokines, which eventually lead to joint pain and swelling. Whether that clinical condition progresses to disability or joint surgery depends on several factors, such as a patient's past medical history and disease severity. Aggressive and early treatment for RA can help, but the effectiveness and accessibility of those interventions can be undermined and limited by low socioeconomic status or poor health behaviors.

Diagnostic Biomarkers

Good clinical criteria for diagnosis of RA do not currently exist, Bathon said. Rather, criteria only exist for RA classification. Because RA is a slowly evolving disease and can take different paths, diagnostic criteria are difficult to develop, she said. But two antibodies are helpful for diagnosis: anti-citrullinated peptide antibody (ACPA) and rheumatoid factor. ACPA has high specificity for RA (more than rheumatoid factor) and has predictive value for the development of RA in a patient who has a positive antibody but no symptoms (Jansen et al., 2002; Nielen et al., 2004; Schellekens et al., 2000). The detection of RA antibodies, however, can precede symptoms by up to 10 years, she added. ACPA is a good diagnostic aid and predictor of downstream disease damage (van Gaalen et al., 2005), but it is not 100 percent specific for RA, she said.

Disease Activity Biomarkers

To assess disease activity, clinicians often rely on a patient self-assessment, a clinical assessment, and the measurement of C-reactive protein. These and other factors combine to form a composite disease activity score, said Bathon. Although there is modest reproducibility in these scores between rheumatologists, there is good reproducibility in the scores if a patient sees the same clinician for serial RA assessment. The strength of assessing the disease activity score is that it can easily be done at clinics for no extra cost, and the scores often correlate with levels of treatment response. Bathon said a laboratory biomarker cannot be substituted for disease activity scores. She added that biomarkers such as C-reactive protein or interleukin-6 are inadequate on their own. There is a commercially available multibiomarker test to measure disease activity for RA called the Vectra DA (Eastman et al., 2012), but questions remain as to whether it is better than clinical disease activity scores for predicting progression of damage on radiograph, she said.

Treatment Response Biomarkers

Treatment response biomarkers include composite scores, radiographic outcomes that can measure the effect of therapy, and patient-reported outcomes, said Bathon. Many modalities used to assess damage or disability in RA do not always correlate with the patient's self-reported pain, but instead they indicate whether or not there is continued joint damage. Understanding whether an RA patient is in remission is also a complex process, using similar composite scores and criteria, she added.

Prognostic Biomarkers

Bathon said that there is not enough data to know whether indicators like radiographically evident joint destruction or high levels of antibodies upon RA diagnosis can predict severity of RA over time. For example, Bathon said a patient with 40 swollen and tender joints may not have more aggressive RA than someone with just two swollen joints. She added that clinicians should try to use all the available biomarkers to assess the patient's risk of "more profound destruction" and treat accordingly.

Finally, Bathon shared that the health assessment questionnaire (HAQ) is the gold standard at FDA for evaluating disability in RA (Buchbinder et al., 1995; Wolfe et al., 2004). The HAQ predicts functional status, work disability, cost of treatment, and more, "so it is a powerful instrument and has been proven to predict RA disease progression," she said (Buchbinder et al., 1995; Pincus et al., 1994; Wolfe et al., 2004). Biomarkers and treatment can help steer patients toward remission and good outcomes, but outcomes are dependent on several factors beyond basic health and biology, Bathon noted.

Osteoarthritis

Kraus provided a brief overview of OA, which can present in the hands, hips, knees, or spine, and can be extremely disabling. All presentations of OA increase with age, and OA often affects women more than men (Murphy et al., 2008; Oliveria et al., 1995). The lifetime risk probability of symptomatic knee OA is approximately 40 percent for men and approximately 47 percent for women, and higher for those who are obese (Murphy et al., 2008).

OA is often associated with pain, fatigue, sleep disturbance, walking disability and inactivity, as well as increased morbidity of heart disease, diabetes, and hypertension (Osteoarthritis Research Society International, 2016). OA is also associated with increased mortality of approximately 55 percent (Osteoarthritis Research Society International, 2016). Early detection of OA can help prevent disability; therefore, biomarkers are critical for OA because pain and imaging changes do not provide an early signal, Kraus emphasized.

Kraus explained that OA affects the entire joint including bone, tissues, joint lining, and articular cartilage. The associated pain comes from collateral damage to other tissues caused by the breakdown of cartilage, she said. Kraus said that CTX-II, a breakdown product of Type II collagen, is the most promising biomarker to date. High baseline CTX-II is associated with a three times higher risk of knee or hip replacement, and a nine times higher risk of knee replacement in the subsequent 2 years (Bjerre-Bastos et al., 2019).

Kraus shared several methods to assess the prognosis of worsening OA. Age and gender, she said, are poorly predictive of worsening OA. However, x-ray is a useful tool, and the more severe the x-ray change, the more likely the individual is to undergo joint replacement (Neogi et al., 2009). Other methods for predicting the risk of worsening OA include a

6-minute walk test (Eyles et al., 2016) and MRI measurements of cartilage loss (Hunter et al., 2011).

To better understand biomarkers in OA, Kraus et al. (2011) had developed their own nomenclature in OA, which preceded the BEST glossary, called BIPEDS, and stands for Burden of disease, Investigational, Prognostic, Efficacy of intervention, Diagnostic biomarkers, and Safety. "While systemic biomarkers can be very useful and report on the whole person, they are not often used in clinical trials because trials are often focused on a single joint with standardized imaging and pain reporting," said Kraus. The challenges for molecular markers of OA are numerous, and the pathogenesis of OA remains complex and multifactorial. Currently, Kraus said, researchers are working on understanding the magnitude of change of a biomarker and how that relates to a clinically meaningful change and outcome in a patient. "Because there are no disease-modifying drugs or treatments for OA, the situation may worsen before it improves" she concluded.

LOW BACK PAIN

Gwendolyn Sowa, chair of the Department of Physical Medicine and Rehabilitation at the University of Pittsburgh, introduced low back pain as a multifactorial condition, similar to other conditions discussed, making it unlikely to use one single biomarker to tell the full story. She noted that the biggest component of disability for back pain comes when the patient transitions from acute to chronic pain. While the most common diagnosis in low back pain is disc degeneration, over time, many more components of the spine are affected than just the intervertebral disc (Vo et al., 2016). As a result, it can be difficult to determine the anatomical identification of the underlying syndrome, even with imaging, she said.

For many years, Sowa said that MRI was the gold standard as a biomarker, but many abnormalities on MRI are not associated with either the patient's symptoms or level of disability. For example, Jensen et al. (1994) found that 52 percent out of 98 asymptomatic people had a disc abnormality. Additionally, lumbar imaging in patients without underlying clinical symptoms does not improve outcomes but does increase incidence of procedures for patients (Chou et al., 2009). Without evidence of improving functional outcomes, the use of this type of traditional imaging as a biomarker is questionable, she asserted. More advanced imaging modalities are in development that may be more clinically useful, but Sowa said they are not ready yet for disability determination.

"Low back pain is a multifactorial syndrome," Sowa reiterated. Current biomarkers fall short because they often are too subjective (e.g., pain scores), not relevant to symptoms (e.g., imaging), or do not correctly assess function, she explained. What is needed, she said, are biomarkers with increased sensitivity to changes of disease activity in real time, and specificity to patient phenotype and individual biology. There is some evidence that circulating biomarkers that are more systemic, such as CTX-II, may provide more insight and prediction of degenerative changes than the existing modalities (Sowa et al., 2009). Protein biomarkers such as neuropeptide Y; regulated on activation, normal T-cell expressed and secreted (RANTES); and CS846 have also demonstrated significant associations with the patient's pain score (Sowa et al., 2014). While individual biomarkers may not provide sufficient information to reflect function, Sowa said that when used in combination they might be more useful than MRI. In addition to the association with pain scores, she said markers such as RANTES, which is a systemic inflammatory biomarker, have been shown to assess functions like gait speed and the Short Performance Physical Battery.

Biomarkers for Treatment

So, Sowa asked, how are biomarkers useful to guide treatment decisions? Biomarkers have been explored for the back pain population in terms of responsiveness to activity (Sowa et al., 2014). It is biologically plausible, and Sowa et al. (2014) have found circulating changes in inflammatory markers respond to activity, which is also associated with function. Regardless of possibilities, she said a one-size-fits-all approach is clearly not going to work for patients with back pain. Many therapies and exercises have been deemed as failures when they likely were not properly titrated to that particular patient and to the patient's disease progression, she added.

Another possibility is using a biomarker to predict the likelihood of response to a specific intervention. A small study was able to identify responders and nonresponders for lumbar epidural steroid injection (Schaaf et al., 2020). The study found that those with improved pain also improved in terms of disability, and the two groups (responders versus nonresponders) showed significant differences in protein biomarkers. She also highlighted genetic biomarkers, which may be relevant to patients with back pain, as emerging evidence shows significant differences in response to treatment between those who carry a certain single nucleotide polymorphism and those who do not (Schaaf et al., 2020).

In closing, Sowa said that low back pain is a syndrome, not a single diagnosis, so determining how to phenotype patients to guide treatment will be an important next step. There is a potential to categorize patients differently based on systemic biomarkers; this would enable testing of treatments that are tailored to a patient's individual needs and help prevent or mitigate the transition from acute to chronic pain and long-term disability, she said.

DISCUSSION

Linda Brady, director of the Division of Neuroscience and Basic Behavioral Science at NIH, and Wallace moderated discussions with the speakers to better understand the translation of their research and clinical findings to be applicable to disability determination. Brady asked about the next steps for biomarkers that have been identified to show early detection in order to develop learning algorithms for predictive treatment outcomes. Etkin said that the next step is validation, with a locked FDA compatible design. While work has been done to validate the tools, there is a need for prospective trials, aligned with what FDA has for an expectation for the biomarker, he explained. Trivedi and Lieberman agreed.

Lieberman elaborated that "once you have a positive indicator of measure, the effort to identify and validate the biomarker will likely be a high-tech next step dependent on academic medical centers." He added that once a biomarker is validated through a sophisticated method, it can be more generalizable. This process of refinement in mental health may take a long time, but "it is not that the pathology is not characterizable, it is just that the technology required has yet to be developed," he shared.

Brady also asked how to best balance the issue of no single biomarker being sufficient to calculate the complexity of a disorder, with the existence of some very simple measures available. Harvey replied that things are "less independent than they seem." Prediction is key, Lieberman said; if genotyping can identify how rare variances play a role in disease progression, then patients could be spared years of medication failures. In the course of illness, it could be possible to predict who becomes severely ill and who responds to treatment, he explained. Trivedi added that both of those scenarios are also present in depression. Some biomarkers could help discern subtypes, but even within subtypes more than one biomarker may be necessary to enhance accuracy of prediction and to be able to match individuals to treatment selection, he said. But that is where he sees the most value; it is still too early for biomarkers for diagnosis of depression.

Rosenbaum asked if the biomarker technologies being discussed are routinely ordered as a standard procedure, and whether insurance would cover them. Lieberman noted that for schizophrenia, biomarkers are not part of a uniform standard of care that is routinely reimbursed, though they are done in some cases. He cautioned that "psychiatry has a checkered past, and we need to be careful about making claims until there is stronger evidence of validation." Trivedi added that reliability of measurement for depression is absolutely accurate, but he suggested part of the reason measurement is not being used is because people have not imagined a new scenario where measurement is routine, and instead they fall back on a basic interview without objective measures. Etkin argued that those who control payment and reimbursement go by what is "standard in the field," and right now most of these technologies are not. He said a more useful question is what value is generated—both clinically and economically—by doing a certain test. He questioned what objective, prespecified targets exist that can determine value for a patient. This type of benchmark for a disease or test "would be a great thing to see," Etkin said.

Rosenbaum also asked about the practical usefulness of this emerging science in the late stage of a disease. By the time someone is so disabled they are applying for disability through SSA, is there a need for some of these more advanced methods and markers, especially when clinical diagnosis and standard procedures are clear, she asked. Clauw noted that by the time someone in pain is contemplating disability, it is very obvious economically and socially, more so than any MRI imaging can determine. Sowa replied that she could see some usefulness for going in the reverse direction—if people are looking to get off of disability, these markers could be useful. Additionally, Kraus said that "OA is increasing so dramatically that there will not be enough joint surgeons to handle the demand," predicting that there will be people in pain who cannot get treatment efficiently due to limited staff and resources.

Thinking about the practicality of biomarkers for SSA, Brady asked which of the biomarkers discussed so far will be cost-effective and practical for use as part of a disability determination interview. Etkin reiterated the need to define value, time, and opportunity, not just cost. Once you have the equipment, he said, EEGs can be done by anyone, and cognitive tests and blood tests are also easy to conduct and cost-effective, so the main question is how good is the biomarker in addressing the value generated through that test. Another view Etkin suggested considering is the perspective of seeing psychiatric disease as a biological disease, and whether there are issues of stigma and compliance. Etkin asked if this will change how patients see themselves and their disease. Trivedi added that "people do not pay enough attention to stigma, and the impact of stigma on a patient's willingness to get diagnosed early." But early diagnosis could really reduce the number of people who need SSA assistance much more than current abilities allow, he said. As a clear and easy incorporation, Harvey said that neuropsychological assessments, some of which only take 30 minutes, can save adjudication in court cases, which is where large amounts of money are often spent.

Wallace asked if emphasis on various radiological biomarkers are causing overmedication or overtreatment, therefore actually increasing disability. Bathon agreed that this can happen. She noted that she has seen this in RA where a patient has pain and after an MRI shows some small erosions, the patient is led down a path of medications and toxicities even if he or she never develops any other pain. Sowa agreed that the same occurs for the low back pain population, where patients "are horrified upon finding out they have degenerative disc disease, but the diagnosis does not give them an understanding of pain, function, or prediction of lifelong disease." From there, she said it is difficult to convince and empower patients that they can get back to work and their activities, and that they should not just rely on a radiographic diagnosis to define their condition.

4

Legal and Ethical Implications

Key Messages from Individual Speakers and Participants

- Determination of disability requires consideration of biological, environmental, and social factors (Bickenbach, Cook, Kirschner).
- The use of biomarkers could exacerbate stigma for diseases that do not have objective findings, making it more difficult for people to recognize a condition in the absence of a marker (Cook, Kirschner).
- Concerns exist for who has access to biomarker information and how that information might be misused (Cook).
- Questions remain as to whether the confidence level in a biomarker is sufficient to determine disability, especially as the biomarker may not fully reflect the patient or their disease, or may even be wrong (Cook, Kirschner, Peterson).
- Individuals may have difficulty interpreting biomarker results, including the clinical implications, and so clinicians and researchers need to carefully consider the best way to disclose this information (Peterson).
- Promising new technologies and findings in medicine may distract health care decision makers from what is most important for people with disabilities to live fully (Bickenbach).

While the emergence of biomarkers offers novel possibilities for prevention, diagnosis, and treatment of difficult diseases, both potential advantages and disadvantages of using biomarkers to determine disability are to be determined. Invited panelists from a variety of backgrounds provided their perspectives in a discussion moderated by Sarah Ruiz, associate director of the Office of Research Sciences at the National Institute on Disability, Independent Living, and Rehabilitation Research. This chapter outlines, from an ethical and legal perspective, the potential benefits and harms of using biomarkers and offers suggestions for SSA as it considers using biomarkers for the determination of disease and disability.

CONCERNS FOR THE USE OF BIOMARKERS IN DISABILITY

With the right supports, Ruiz said, "people with disabilities can participate fully in society. Yet, we know that entrenched ableism and discrimination against people with disabilities is a longstanding challenge and barrier to full participation." As we consider the legal and ethical implications of the use of biomarkers, she said, it is important to take a holistic, even macro approach in our concerns. Disability is not just about the individual—it can also affect families, communities, and society. During their remarks, panelists covered both the potential harms and benefits of SSA using biomarkers to assist in disability determination.

Jerome Bickenbach, professor of law in the Department of Health Sciences and Medicine at the University of Lucerne, described much of his work with former Soviet countries to move away from a purely medical approach to one that identifies disability as a clear function of the environmental context in which a person lives. In other words, he said, while a medical determination is crucial for a disease diagnosis and prognosis, it often has nothing to do with a disability assessment. In the countries he works with, the goal has become to more fully integrate disability assessment into overall disability policy more seamlessly and regard the individual's environmental context as a series of assets that can be built to fully include the person in society. For example, you would not assess someone with paraplegia without considering their wheelchair, he said.

Judith Cook, director of the Center on Mental Health Services Research and Policy at the University of Illinois at Chicago, added that the social model of disability asserts that the same types and levels of impairment in different people may or may not be disabling due to a variety of factors. She said that people with high levels of psychiatric symptoms may be able to work their entire lives in a job that provides accommodations and a supportive social environment, so the use of biomarkers to truly predict disability will require biological, environmental, and social factors. Big data may be helpful in modeling these complex associations, but she cautioned against an oversimplified application of mental illness biomarkers.

Cook added that the use of biomarkers in this determination process could actually increase objectivity and reduce the subjectivity of judgements about whether a person has a disabling mental health condition. Kristi Kirschner, clinical professor at the University of Illinois College of Medicine, highlighted that many chronic fatigue patients live with incredible pain and significant disability, but they lack objective findings, which contributes to their stigma and shame because people often ask if the conditions are real. Kirschner was concerned that biomarkers could exacerbate the disparities between diseases that have objective findings and those that do not, making it more difficult for people to recognize a condition even in the absence of a marker.

Andrew Peterson, assistant professor of philosophy and public policy at George Mason University, shared his research on patients who have experienced traumatic brain injuries resulting in comas and required the use of assessment tools to understand prognosis (Peterson and Bayne, 2018; Peterson et al., 2015, 2020a). More recently, he and his colleagues have explored biomarkers in Alzheimer's to identify clinical signs of cognitive decline even if a patient has been asymptomatic for years (Largent et al., 2019, 2020). "So how do you tell patients this," he asked, and added, "What is the right way to disclose this sensitive information?" He said, "biomarkers can be really difficult for patients to process and understand upon exposure." Clinicians and researchers need to carefully consider the best way to disclose this information (Mozersky et al., 2018; Peterson et al., 2020b), he added. Another consideration he shared, which echoed other panelists, is that biomarkers can be both stigmatizing and empowering at the same time. The relationship between biomarkers and stigma is complex, he emphasized.

POTENTIAL HARMS AND BENEFITS

A few speakers cautioned about potential harms for using biomarkers. Cook noted that some of the medical conditions discussed are associated with high levels of social stigma, including in hiring and employment. She referenced literature citing concerns of who has access to biomarker information and how that information might be misused (Jurjako et al., 2018; Lakhan et al., 2010; Lehrner and Yehuda, 2014; Rothenberger et al., 2015). There is also controversy in certain illnesses, such as PTSD or major depression, about people exaggerating the effects of mental illnesses on their functional capacity—malingering, she said. She said evidence suggests that the predictive validity of self-perception is important to include in models; Davillas and Pudney (2020) found the effects of biomarkers as disability predictors dropped by a range of 20 to 40 percent when the person's self-assessed health was introduced to the model.

Cook noted that it is very difficult to define the level of confidence for a biomarker, and asked who decides when the confidence level is strong enough in disability determination or continuing review. Peterson added that there is a need to acknowledge the risk of being wrong within the biomarker system. Similar to discussions in Chapter 3, Kirschner worried that people may rely too much on biomarkers to learn about the disease and the patient rather than what the biomarker is capable of, especially for people without health insurance or low levels of health literacy.

CONSIDERATIONS FOR DECISION MAKING IN DEFINING DISABILITY

"Disability is a complex interactive phenomenon that has biological, social, and contextual elements," said Kirschner. While some patients with disabilities have clear objective findings to document their conditions, disease categories are reductive, she said, and we want to understand the lived experience of the disease in a person. Rosenbaum commented that the definition of disability that SSA has to grapple with requires establishing that there is an impairment that can be named. It also requires proving that impairment prevents an individual from being able to engage in substantial activity. She asked the panelists what considerations SSA may have for both of these issues. Kirschner replied that "in the absence of objective data, we are in the realm of clinical diagnosis, and within the SSA system, there is no lab test or X-ray available," so she called for embracing the limitations of our knowledge. Lieberman suggested that if someone has a condition that lacks confirmation, yet has clinical credibility, that might be sufficient. He asked if SSA could track longitudinal disease course and outcomes for these types of patients to ensure monitoring, similar to how insurance companies follow people to ensure no fraud is committed.

Bickenbach called attention to the issue of multiple morbidities. Individually certain diseases may not be too bad, but when combined, the sum is greater than the whole of the parts in terms of the overall effect on life, he said. A person may not have a condition or disability that meets the threshold, he said, but they have lives that are unlivable because they are dealing with so many conditions at once. Cook suggested that the use of biomarkers for disability determination needs to occur in the context of an interdisciplinary discussion that includes people with disabilities who can help inform how the intersecting social model of disability and biological model of disability work to influence important life functions.

Finally, Bickenbach noted that the concern in the disability field is that new technologies and findings in medicine may divert attention from what is actually needed and emphasized that anything being explored should be fit for its purpose. In Europe, there is an increasing focus on integration and a participatory role—understanding what can help people live their lives more fully, he said.

5

Final Thoughts

Key Messages from Individual Speakers and Participants

- The connections between currently validated biomarkers and the progression of these diseases and conditions to a level of disability that prevents an individual from engaging in substantial gainful activity as understood under the Social Security law remains tenuous (Diamond, Morris, Rosenbaum, Shoulson).
- One of the important factors for integrating biomarkers is to know the risks of being wrong—to both the individual and society (Diamond, Peterson).
- A continued challenge will be translating findings from a cohort or subgroup to an individual for disability determination (Morris, Rosenbaum).
- Diversity (e.g., race, gender, age, disabilities) should be ensured in biomarker studies to avoid incorrectly assuming a "one-size-fits-all" approach and potentially exacerbating health disparities (Nitkin).
- In most cases, biomarker research is a long way from clinical application (Shoulson).

A variety of different types of biomarkers are present in individuals over the course of their disease process. The emerging research that informs clinical understanding and application of these biomarkers for diagnosis and prognosis of disease, as well as more personalized treatment regimens, is exciting. However, the connections between currently validated biomarkers and the progression of these diseases and conditions to a level of disability that prevents an individual from engaging in substantial gainful activity as understood under the Social Security law remains tenuous. This chapter summarizes the positive findings and potential uses of biomarkers, as well as their challenges from several perspectives. Finally, it offers considerations to SSA for incorporating biomarkers in its process for determination of disability.

EXAMINING POSITIVE FINDINGS AND POTENTIAL CHALLENGES

In reaction to the discussions throughout the workshop, a panel made up of several members of the workshop planning committee shared the key points they heard in terms of the state of the science and the possible challenges that lay ahead as biomarkers continue to be developed. The panel included Betty Diamond, director of the Institute of Molecular Medicine at the Feinstein Institutes for Medical Research; Sarah Morris, chief of the Adult Psychopathology and Psychosocial Intervention Research Branch at the National Institutes of Mental Health; Ralph Nitkin, deputy director for the National Center for Medical Rehabilitation Research at NIH's National Institute of Child Health and Human Development; and Ira Shoulson, professor of neurology, pharmacology, and medicine at the University of Rochester School of Medicine.

Potential Use of Biomarkers

Various types of biomarkers were highlighted throughout the workshop, including molecular, chemical, and systemic—showing the breadth of potential biomarkers that researchers can study when looking for indicators to assist in more accurate diagnostic, prognostic, or treatment determinations. Shoulson commented that the whole field of biomarkers has immediate and long-term application to disease—both related to diagnosis and prognosis. Prognostic biomarkers, especially, could be very valuable in determining the outlook for a person, he said.

Nitkin noted the importance of a functional goal for biomarkers, saying biomarkers need to be useful, whether it is to do things more quickly or in different environments (e.g., at point-of-care instead of limited to certain lab capacity), or to offer more predictive or precise care for patients. He acknowledged "disability rehabilitation is a tricky field" because it is contextually and environmentally dependent. Morris emphasized the importance of research that capitalizes on big data—such as data already available in electronic medical records that do not require a lot of new expertise or equipment.

Continued Challenges

Diamond called attention to the potential for being wrong, asking what are the risks to individuals or to society? This comment also echoed Peterson's previous remarks about the need to grapple with the risk of false positives and false negatives and understand what the risk of being wrong with biomarker assessment will be in a clinical context or in a disability application. To help understand the risks of biomarkers, Diamond agreed with Menetski, saying systemic redefinition of terms may be needed. For example, is SSA trying to identify people who can or cannot work, or just determine what services and supports are needed to make that person a more productive member of society, she asked.

Morris reiterated the disconnect between approaches to research and the challenge of making a disability determination that Rosenbaum raised, which exists because most research studies are focused on comparing a group of patients with a group of comparison subjects. Studies also may sometimes identify subgroups within a sample of participants and discover relationships between brain and behavior and functioning. However, Morris said, the gaps in research become obvious when an agency, like SSA, asks what the cutoff is for certain markers. She said the current research findings

> do not necessarily translate nicely into informing a dichotomous disability determination that has to be made on the basis of one individual tested in isolation, compared to the context of a whole group of research participants, which is where the findings originated.

She noted the burden would be on SSA to weigh what acceptable rates of false positives and false negatives would be. To address the research side, Morris called for better standardized tests and measures that can be used and interpreted for one individual in each site. Finally, Shoulson pointed out that most of the research presented was informative, but it currently seems emerging at best, and thus it is a long way from clinical application.

SUGGESTIONS FOR THE USE OF BIOMARKERS IN THE SOCIAL SECURITY ADMINISTRATION

As biomarkers are validated, Nitkin said, they are typically based on retrospective studies and populations that are often representing the majority and are easily accessible. But the results of those studies should not be applied to the generalized population, he cautioned. Lack of diversity in studies could inadvertently cause health disparities by using biomarkers too broadly, he said.

Shoulson noted that what patients report (e.g., patient-reported outcomes) of their symptoms alone accounts for approximately 80 percent of accurate diagnoses—as agreed upon by experienced, expert clinicians. So, this "low-hanging fruit" offers an opportunity, he added. Using tools and technology such as machine learning, he said, and by listening to patients and pairing their subjective reports with objective clinical information can help clinicians further determine a patient's disease progress. Shoulson also thought it would be useful if biomarkers related highly to function. He suggested exploring and examining this connection more closely—especially in relation to gainful activity—to understand how to make a better determination for people using that lens.

References

All of Us Research Program Investigators. 2019. The "All of Us" research program. *New England Journal of Medicine* 381(7):668–676.

Bjerre-Bastos, J., A.-C. Bay-Jensen, M. Karsdal, I. Byrjalsen, J. R. Andersen, B. J. Riis, C. Christiansen, and A. R. Bihlet. 2019. THU0419 biomarkers of bone and cartilage turnover CTX-I and CTX-II predict total joint replacements in OA. *Annals of the Rheumatic Diseases* 78(Suppl 2):497–498.

Brummett, C. M., A. G. Urquhart, A. L. Hassett, A. Tsodikov, B. R. Hallstrom, N. I. Wood, D. A. Williams, and D. J. Clauw. 2015. Characteristics of fibromyalgia independently predict poorer long-term analgesic outcomes following total knee and hip arthroplasty. *Arthritis Rheumatoly* 67(5):1386–1394.

Buchbinder, R., C. Bombardier, M. Yeung, and P. Tugwell. 1995. Which outcome measures should be used in rheumatoid arthritis clinical trials? *Arthritis & Rheumatism* 38(11):1568–1580.

Cassidy, C. M., F. A. Zucca, R. R. Girgis, S. C. Baker, J. J. Weinstein, M. E. Sharp, C. Bellei, A. Valmadre, N. Vanegas, L. S. Kegeles, G. Brucato, U. J. Kang, D. Sulzer, L. Zecca, A. Abi-Dargham, and G. Horga. 2019. Neuromelanin-sensitive MRI as a noninvasive proxy measure of dopamine function in the human brain. *Proceedings of the National Academy of Sciences* 116(11):5108–5117.

CDER (Center for Drug Evaluation and Research). 2018. *Biomarker qualification: Evidentiary framework.* https://www.fda.gov/media/119271/download (accessed September 3, 2020).

Chou, R., R. Fu, J. A. Carrino, and R. A. Deyo. 2009. Imaging strategies for low-back pain: Systematic review and meta-analysis. *Lancet* 373(9662):463–472.

Collins, F. S., and H. Varmus. 2015. A new initiative on precision medicine. *New England Journal of Medicine* 372(9):793–795.

Davillas, A., and S. Pudney. 2020. Biomarkers as precursors of disability. *Economics & Human Biology* 36:100814.

Depp, C. A., J. Bashem, R. C. Moore, J. L. Holden, T. Mikhael, J. Swendsen, P. D. Harvey, and E. L. Granholm. 2019. GPS mobility as a digital biomarker of negative symptoms in schizophrenia: A case control study. *NPJ Digital Medicine* 2(1):108.

Eastman, P. S., W. C. Manning, F. Qureshi, D. Haney, G. Cavet, C. Alexander, and L. K. Hesterberg. 2012. Characterization of a multiplex, 12-biomarker test for rheumatoid arthritis. *Journal of Pharmaceutical and Biomedical Analysis* 70:415–424.

Eyles, J. P., K. Mills, B. R. Lucas, M. J. Williams, J. Makovey, L. Teoh, and D. J. Hunter. 2016. Can we predict those with osteoarthritis who will worsen following a chronic disease management program? *Arthritis Care and Research* 68(9):1268–1277.

FDA-NIH (Food and Drug Administration-National Institutes of Health) Biomarker Working Group. 2016 *BEST (biomarkers, endpoints, and other tools) resource*. Silver Spring, MD: Food and Drug Administration.

FNIH (Foundation for the National Institutes of Health). 2020. *About the biomarkers consortium*. https://fnih.org/what-we-do/biomarkers-consortium/about (accessed September 25, 2020).

Fonzo, G. A., A. Etkin, Y. Zhang, W. Wu, C. Cooper, C. Chin-Fatt, M. K. Jha, J. Trombello, T. Deckersbach, P. Adams, M. McInnis, P. J. McGrath, M. M. Weissman, M. Fava, and M. H. Trivedi. 2019. Brain regulation of emotional conflict predicts antidepressant treatment response for depression. *Nature Human Behaviour* 3(12):1319–1331.

Granholm, E., J. L. Holden, T. Mikhael, P. C. Link, J. Swendsen, C. Depp, R. C. Moore, and P. D. Harvey. 2020. What do people with schizophrenia do all day? Ecological momentary assessment of real-world functioning in schizophrenia. *Schizophrenia Bulletin* 46(2):242–251.

Harvey, P. D., R. K. Heaton, W. T. Carpenter, Jr., M. F. Green, J. M. Gold, and M. Schoenbaum. 2012. Functional impairment in people with schizophrenia: Focus on employability and eligibility for disability compensation. *Schizophrenia Research* 140(1–3):1–8.

Hunter, D. J., W. Zhang, P. G. Conaghan, K. Hirko, L. Menashe, W. M. Reichmann, and E. Losina. 2011. Responsiveness and reliability of MRI in knee osteoarthritis: A meta-analysis of published evidence. *Osteoarthritis Cartilage* 19(5):589–605.

Janda, A. M., S. As-Sanie, B. Rajala, A. Tsodikov, S. E. Moser, D. J. Clauw, and C. M. Brummett. 2015. Fibromyalgia survey criteria are associated with increased postoperative opioid consumption in women undergoing hysterectomy. *Anesthesiology* 122(5):1103–1111.

Jansen, A. L., I. van der Horst-Bruinsma, D. van Schaardenburg, R. J. van de Stadt, M. H. de Koning, and B. A. Dijkmans. 2002. Rheumatoid factor and antibodies to cyclic citrullinated peptide differentiate rheumatoid arthritis from undifferentiated polyarthritis in patients with early arthritis. *Journal of Rheumatolgy* 29(10):2074–2076.

Jensen, M. C., M. N. Brant-Zawadzki, N. Obuchowski, M. T. Modic, D. Malkasian, and J. S. Ross. 1994. Magnetic resonance imaging of the lumbar spine in people without back pain. *New England Journal of Medicine* 331(2):69–73.

Jha, M. K., A. Minhajuddin, B. S. Gadad, T. Greer, B. Grannemann, A. Soyombo, T. L. Mayes, A. J. Rush, and M. H. Trivedi. 2017. Can C-reactive protein inform antidepressant medication selection in depressed outpatients? Findings from the CO-MED trial. *Psychoneuroendocrinology* 78:105–113.

Jurjako, M., L. Malatesti, and I. A. Brazil. 2019. Some ethical considerations about the use of biomarkers for the classification of adult antisocial individuals. *International Journal of Forensic Mental Health* 18(3):228–242.

Keefe, R. S., M. Poe, T. M. Walker, J. W. Kang, and P. D. Harvey. 2006. The schizophrenia cognition rating scale: An interview-based assessment and its relationship to cognition, real-world functioning, and functional capacity. *American Journal of Psychiatry* 163(3):426–432.

REFERENCES

Keren, H., G. O'Callaghan, P. Vidal-Ribas, G. A. Buzzell, M. A. Brotman, E. Leibenluft, P. M. Pan, L. Meffert, A. Kaiser, S. Wolke, D. S. Pine, and A. Stringaris. 2018. Reward processing in depression: A conceptual and meta-analytic review across FMRI and EEG studies. *American Journal of Psychiatry* 175(11):1111–1120.

Kraus, V. B., B. Burnett, J. Coindreau, S. Cottrell, D. Eyre, M. Gendreau, J. Gardiner, P. Garnero, J. Hardin, Y. Henrotin, D. Heinegård, A. Ko, L. S. Lohmander, G. Matthews, J. Menetski, R. Moskowitz, S. Persiani, A. R. Poole, J. C. Rousseau, M. Todman, and OARSI FDA Osteoarthritis Biomarkers Working Group. 2011. Application of biomarkers in the development of drugs intended for the treatment of osteoarthritis. *Osteoarthritis and Cartilage* 19(5):515–542.

Lakhan, S. E., K. Vieira, and E. Hamlat. 2010. Biomarkers in psychiatry: Drawbacks and potential for misuse. *International Archives of Medicine* 3:1.

Largent, E. A., M. Terrasse, K. Harkins, D. A. Sisti, P. Sankar, and J. Karlawish. 2019. Attitudes toward physician-assisted death from individuals who learn they have an Alzheimer disease biomarker. *JAMA Neurology* 76(7):864–866.

Largent, E. A., K. Harkins, C. H. van Dyck, S. Hachey, P. Sankar, and J. Karlawish. 2020. Cognitively unimpaired adults' reactions to disclosure of amyloid PET scan results. *PloS One* 15(2):e0229137.

Laruelle, M., L. S. Kegeles, and A. Abi-Dargham. 2003. Glutamate, dopamine, and schizophrenia. *Annals of the New York Academy of Sciences* 1003(1):138–158.

Lehrner, A., and R. Yehuda. 2014. Biomarkers of PTSD: Military applications and considerations. *European Journal of Psychotraumatology* 5:10.3402/ejpt.v3405.23797.

Leptak, C., J. P. Menetski, J. A. Wagner, J. Aubrecht, L. Brady, M. Brumfield, W. W. Chin, S. Hoffmann, G. Kelloff, G. Lavezzari, R. Ranganathan, J. M. Sauer, F. D. Sistare, T. Zabka, and D. Wholley. 2017. What evidence do we need for biomarker qualification? *Science Translational Medicine* 9(417).

López-Solà, M., C.-W. Woo, J. Pujol, J. Deus, B. J. Harrison, J. Monfort, and T. D. Wager. 2017. Towards a neurophysiological signature for fibromyalgia. *Pain* 158(1):34–47.

Maixner, W., R. B. Fillingim, D. A. Williams, S. B. Smith, and G. D. Slade. 2016. Overlapping chronic pain conditions: Implications for diagnosis and classification. *Journal of Pain* 17(9 Suppl):T93–T107.

Menetski, J. P., S. C. Hoffmann, S. S. Cush, T. N. Kamphaus, C. P. Austin, P. L. Herrling, and J. A. Wagner. 2019. The Foundation for the National Institutes of Health Biomarkers Consortium: Past accomplishments and new strategic direction. *Clinical Pharmacology & Therapeutics* 105(4):829–843.

Milleville, K., R. G. Kumar, D. Disanto, and A. K. Wagner. 2019. Post-acute systemic inflammatory biomarkers and cognition after TBI: A follow-up study. *Journal of Neurotrauma* 36(13):A123.

Mozersky, J., P. Sankar, K. Harkins, S. Hachey, and J. Karlawish. 2018. Comprehension of an elevated amyloid positron emission tomography biomarker result by cognitively normal older adults. *JAMA Neurology* 75(1):44–50.

Murphy, L., T. A. Schwartz, C. G. Helmick, J. B. Renner, G. Tudor, G. Koch, A. Dragomir, W. D. Kalsbeek, G. Luta, and J. M. Jordan. 2008. Lifetime risk of symptomatic knee osteoarthritis. *Arthritis Care & Research* 59(9):1207–1213.

Neogi, T., D. Felson, J. Niu, M. Nevitt, C. E. Lewis, P. Aliabadi, B. Sack, J. Torner, L. Bradley, and Y. Zhang. 2009. Association between radiographic features of knee osteoarthritis and pain: Results from two cohort studies. *British Journal of Management* 339:b2844.

Nielen, M. M., D. van Schaardenburg, H. W. Reesink, R. J. van de Stadt, I. E. van der Horst-Bruinsma, M. H. de Koning, M. R. Habibuw, J. P. Vandenbroucke, and B. A. Dijkmans. 2004. Specific autoantibodies precede the symptoms of rheumatoid arthritis: A study of serial measurements in blood donors. *Arthritis and Rheumatism* 50(2):380–386.

Oliveria, S. A., D. T. Felson, J. I. Reed, P. A. Cirillo, and A. M. Walker. 1995. Incidence of symptomatic hand, hip, and knee osteoarthritis among patients in a health maintenance organization. *Arthritis and Rheumatism* 38(8):1134–1141.

Osimo, E. F., T. Pillinger, I. M. Rodriguez, G. M. Khandaker, C. M. Pariante, and O. D. Howes. 2020. Inflammatory markers in depression: A meta-analysis of mean differences and variability in 5,166 patients and 5,083 controls. *Brain, Behavior, and Immunity* 87:901–909.

Osteoarthritis Research Society International. 2016. *Osteoarthritis: A serious disease.* Submitted to the Food and Drug Administration.

Peterson, A., and T. Bayne. 2018. Post-comatose disorders of consciousness. In *The Routledge handbook of consciousness*, edited by R. J. Gennaro. New York: Taylor & Francis.

Peterson, A., D. Cruse, L. Naci, C. Weijer, and A. M. Owen. 2015. Risk, diagnostic error, and the clinical science of consciousness. *NeuroImage Clinical* 7:588–597.

Peterson, A., A. M. Owen, and J. Karlawish. 2020a. Alive inside. *Bioethics* 34(3):295–305.

Peterson, A., A. M. Owen, and J. Karlawish. 2020b. Translating the discovery of covert consciousness into clinical practice. *JAMA Neurology* 77(5):541–542.

Pincus, T., R. H. Brooks, and L. F. Callahan. 1994. Prediction of long-term mortality in patients with rheumatoid arthritis according to simple questionnaire and joint count measures. *Annals Internal Medicine* 120(1):26–34.

Raugh, I. M., S. H. James, C. M. Gonzalez, H. C. Chapman, A. S. Cohen, B. Kirkpatrick, and G. P. Strauss. 2020. Geolocation as a digital phenotyping measure of negative symptoms and functional outcome. *Schizophrenia Bulletin* 121.

Robinson, D. G., M. G. Woerner, M. McMeniman, A. Mendelowitz, and R. M. Bilder. 2004. Symptomatic and functional recovery from a first episode of schizophrenia or schizoaffective disorder. *American Journal of Psychiatry* 161(3):473–479.

Roth, M., B. E. Tomlinson, and G. Blessed. 1967. The relationship between quantitative measures of dementia and of degenerative changes in the cerebral grey matter of elderly subjects. *Proceedings of the Royal Society of Medicine* 60(3):254–260.

Rothenberger, A., L. A. Rhode, and L. G. Rothenberger. 2015. Biomarkers in child mental health: A bio-psycho-social perspective is needed. *Behavioral and Brain Functions* 11(1):31.

Sartorius, N. 2006. The meanings of health and its promotion. *Croatian Medical Journal* 47(4):662–664.

Schaaf, S., W. Huang, S. Perera, Y. Conley, I. Belfer, P. Jayabalan, K. Tremont, P. Coelho, S. Ernst, M. Cortazzo, D. Weiner, D., N. Vo, J. Kang, and G. Sowa. 2020. Association of protein and genetic biomarkers with response to lumbar epidural steroid injections in subjects with axial low back pain. *American Journal of Physical Medicine and Rehabilitation*. Online ahead of print.

Schellekens, G. A., H. Visser, B. A. de Jong, F. H. van den Hoogen, J. M. Hazes, F. C. Breedveld, and W. J. van Venrooij. 2000. The diagnostic properties of rheumatoid arthritis antibodies recognizing a cyclic citrullinated peptide. *Arthritis and Rheumatism* 43(1):155–163.

Sowa, G., E. Westrick, A. Rajasekhar, B. Woods, S. Leckie, N. Vo, R. Studer, and J. Kang. 2009. Identification of candidate serum biomarkers for intervertebral disk degeneration in an animal model. *PM&R: The Journal of Injury, Function, and Rehabilitation* 536–540.

Sowa, G. A., S. Perera, B. Bechara, V. Agarwal, J. Boardman, W. Huang, A. Camacho-Soto, N. Vo, J. Kang, and D. Weiner. 2014. Associations between serum biomarkers and pain and pain-related function in older adults with low back pain: A pilot study. *Journal of American Geriatric Society* 62(11):2047–2055.

REFERENCES

SSA (Social Security Administration). 2020. *Disability evaulation under Social Security.* https://www.ssa.gov/disability/professionals/bluebook/general-info.htm (accessed September 1, 2020).

Stein, P. 2020. *Brief overview of biomarkers: Value, limitations, and the Biomarker Qualification Program (BQP).* https://fnih.org/sites/default/files/final/pdf/2-Stein-Biomarkers%20Introduction.pdf (accessed September 21, 2020).

Strassnig, M., D. Cornacchio, P. D. Harvey, R. Kotov, L. Fochtmann, and E. J. Bromet. 2017a. Health status and mobility limitations are associated with residential and employment status in schizophrenia and bipolar disorder. *Journal of Psychiatric Research* 94:180–185.

Strassnig, M., R. Kotov, D. Cornaccio, L. Fochtmann, P. D. Harvey, and E. J. Bromet. 2017b. Twenty-year progression of body mass index in a county-wide cohort of people with schizophrenia and bipolar disorder identified at their first episode of psychosis. *Bipolar Disorder* 19(5):336–343.

Sulzer, D., J. Bogulavsky, K. E. Larsen, G. Behr, E. Karatekin, M. H. Kleinman, N. Turro, D. Krantz, R. H. Edwards, L. A. Greene, and L. Zecca. 2000. Neuromelanin biosynthesis is driven by excess cytosolic catecholamines not accumulated by synaptic vesicles. *Proceedings of the National Academy of Sciences* 97(22):11869–11874.

Trivedi, M. H., T. L. Greer, T. S. Church, T. J. Carmody, B. D. Grannemann, D. I. Galper, A. L. Dunn, C. P. Earnest, P. Sunderajan, S. S. Henley, and S. N. Blair. 2011. Exercise as an augmentation treatment for nonremitted major depressive disorder: A randomized, parallel dose comparison. *Journal of Clinical Psychiatry* 72(5):677–684.

VA (Department of Veterans Affairs). 2020. *Million Veteran Program.* https://www.mvp.va.gov/webapp/mvp-web-participant/#/public (accessed September 24, 2020).

van Gaalen, F. A., H. Visser, and T. W. J. Huizinga. 2005. A comparison of the diagnostic accuracy and prognostic value of the first and second anti-cyclic citrullinated peptides (CCP1 and CCP2) autoantibody tests for rheumatoid arthritis. *Annals of the Rheumatic Diseases* 64(10):1510–1512.

Ventura, J., K. L. Subotnik, M. J. Gitlin, D. Gretchen-Doorly, A. Ered, K. F. Villa, G. S. Hellemann, and K. H. Nuechterlein. 2015. Negative symptoms and functioning during the first year after a recent onset of schizophrenia and 8 years later. *Schizophrenia Research* 161(2–3):407–413.

Ventura, J., K. L. Subotnik, D. Gretchen-Doorly, L. Casaus, M. Boucher, A. Medalia, M. D. Bell, G. S. Hellemann, and K. H. Nuechterlein. 2019. Cognitive remediation can improve negative symptoms and social functioning in first-episode schizophrenia: A randomized controlled trial. *Schizophrenia Research* 203:24–31.

Vo, N. V., R. A. Hartman, P. R. Patil, M. V. Risbud, D. Kletsas, J. C. Iatridis, J. A. Hoyland, C. L. Le Maitre, G. A. Sowa, and J. D. Kang. 2016. Molecular mechanisms of biological aging in intervertebral discs. *Journal of Orthopaedic Research* 34(8):1289–1306.

WHO (World Health Organization). 2001. *International classification of functioning disability and health.* https://www.who.int/classifications/icf/en (accessed September 8, 2020).

WHO. 2002. *Towards a common language for functioning, disability and health.* https://www.who.int/classifications/icf/training/icfbeginnersguide.pdf (accessed October 1, 2020).

Wolfe, F., K. Michaud, and T. Pincus. 2004. Development and validation of the health assessment questionnaire II: A revised version of the health assessment questionnaire. *Arthritis & Rheumatism* 50(10):3296–3305.

Wu, W., Y. Zhang, J. Jiang, M. V.Lucas, G. A. Fonzo, C. E. Rolle, C. Cooper, C. Chin-Fatt, N. Krepel, C. A. Cornelssen, R. Wright, R. T. Toll, H. M. Trivedi, K. Monuszko, T. L. Caudle, M. K. Sarhadi, J. M. Trombello, T. Deckersbach, P. Adams, P. J. McGrath, M. M. Weissman, M. Fava D. A. Pizzagalli, M. Arns, M. H, Trivedi, and A. Etkin. 2020. An electroencephalographic signature predicts antidepressant response in major depression. *Nature Biotechnology* 38(4):439–447.

Zhang, Y., W. Wu, R. T. Toll, S. Naparstek, A. Maron-Katz, M. Watts, J. Gordon, J. Jeong, L. Astolfi, E. Shpigel, P. Longwell, K. Sarhadi, D. El-Said, Y. Li, C. Cooper, C. Chin-Fatt, M. Arns, M. S. Goodkind, M. H. Trivedi, C. R. Marmar, and A. Etkin. 2020. Identification of psychiatric disorder subtypes from functional connectivity patterns in resting-state electroencephalography. *Nature Biomedical Engineering*. Epub ahead of print.

Appendix A

Statement of Task

The National Academies of Sciences, Engineering, and Medicine shall establish an ad hoc planning committee to plan and host a 1- to 2-day public workshop to facilitate a discussion focused on the use of biomarkers to establish the presence and severity of disability.

The meeting will feature invited presentations and discussions on topics such as:

1. A general overview of biomarkers and the current and potential purposes for their use, including presentations which explain:
   a. The accuracy of the definitions of key terms in biomarker research, to be provided by the Social Security Administration (e.g., *clinical endpoint, surrogate endpoint, telomere*);
   b. The difference between the term "biomarker" (which may include traits or metrics such as height or blood pressure) from the more specific "molecular biomarker" for which the term is typically used as an abbreviation;
   c. The types of diagnostic, non-genetic biomarkers (e.g., distinct anatomical or physiological signatures); and
   d. The range of impairments for which health care professionals currently use diagnostic and prognostic biomarkers and their potential for use in the future.
2. How health care professionals now use non-genetic biomarkers as diagnostic/prognostic tools and severity indicators in the following physical and mental impairments (whether as a sole indicator

of the presence of impairment or as confirmation of a clinically significant sign associated with the impairment), and summarize the supporting research:
   a. Fibromyalgia;
   b. Arthritis;
   c. Post-traumatic stress disorder;
   d. Major depression;
   e. Schizophrenia; and
   f. Chronic pain.
3. Whether it is typical for health care professionals to:
   a. Associate any biomarker with a particular level of functional status; and
   b. Use any biomarker as a sole indicator of impairment severity.
4. The legal and ethical implications associated with biomarker use in clinical decision making.

A proceedings of the presentations and discussions at the workshop will be prepared by a designated rapporteur in accordance with institutional guidelines.

Appendix B

Workshop Agenda

JULY 21, 2020

10:00 a.m. **Welcome and Opening Remarks**
SARA ROSENBAUM, *THE GEORGE WASHINGTON UNIVERSITY PLANNING COMMITTEE CHAIR*

Sponsor Remarks from the Social Security Administration
MARK WARSHAWSKY, *SOCIAL SECURITY ADMINISTRATION*

10:15 a.m. **Session 1: Overview of Biomarkers**
Moderator: SARA ROSENBAUM, *THE GEORGE WASHINGTON UNIVERSITY*

Overview of Terminology and Biomarker Use in Clinical Decision Making
JOSEPH MENETSKI, *FOUNDATION FOR THE NATIONAL INSTITUTES OF HEALTH*

Where Do Biomarkers Fit When Trying to Relate Health to Function?
AMY WAGNER, *UNIVERSITY OF PITTSBURGH*

	Panel Discussion
11:15 a.m.	**Break**
11:30 a.m.	**Session 2: Bioethical and Legal Considerations with the Use of Biomarkers to Establish Presence and Severity of Impairments** **Moderator:** SARAH RUIZ, NATIONAL INSTITUTE ON DISABILITY, INDEPENDENT LIVING, AND REHABILITATION RESEARCH
	Panelists JEROME BICKENBACH, UNIVERSITY OF LUCERNE JUDITH COOK, UNIVERSITY OF ILLINOIS AT CHICAGO CENTER ON MENTAL HEALTH SERVICES RESEARCH AND POLICY KRISTI KIRSCHNER, UNIVERSITY OF ILLINOIS COLLEGE OF MEDICINE ANDREW PETERSON, GEORGE MASON UNIVERSITY
	Panel Discussion
12:15 p.m.	**Lunch Break**
12:45 p.m.	**Session 3: State of the Science on Biomarkers to Establish Presence and Severity of Impairments: Part I** (major depression, post-traumatic stress disorder, and schizophrenia) **Moderator:** LINDA BRADY, NATIONAL INSTITUTES OF HEALTH
	Panelists MADHUKAR TRIVEDI, UNIVERSITY OF TEXAS SOUTHWESTERN MEDICAL CENTER AT DALLAS AMIT ETKIN, STANFORD UNIVERSITY AND ALTO NEUROSCIENCE JEFFREY LIEBERMAN, COLUMBIA UNIVERSITY PHILIP HARVEY, UNIVERSITY OF MIAMI
	Panel Discussion
2:20 p.m.	**Break**

2:35 p.m.	**Session 3: State of the Science on Biomarkers to Establish Presence and Severity of Impairments: Part II** (arthritis, chronic pain, and fibromyalgia) **Moderator:** ROBERT WALLACE, UNIVERSITY OF IOWA **Panelists** DANIEL CLAUW, UNIVERSITY OF MICHIGAN JOAN BATHON, COLUMBIA UNIVERSITY VIRGINIA BYERS KRAUS, DUKE MOLECULAR PHYSIOLOGY INSTITUTE GWENDOLYN SOWA, UNIVERSITY OF PITTSBURGH **Panel Discussion**
4:15 p.m.	**Session 5: Reactor Panel** **Moderator:** SARA ROSENBAUM, THE GEORGE WASHINGTON UNIVERSITY **Panelists** BETTY DIAMOND, HOFSTRA NORTHWELL SCHOOL OF MEDICINE SARAH MORRIS, NATIONAL INSTITUTES OF HEALTH RALPH NITKIN, NATIONAL INSTITUTES OF HEALTH IRA SHOULSON, UNIVERSITY OF ROCHESTER
4:45 p.m.	**Public Comment**
4:55 p.m.	**Workshop Wrap-Up** SARA ROSENBAUM, THE GEORGE WASHINGTON UNIVERSITY PLANNING COMMITTEE CHAIR
5:00 p.m.	**Adjourn**

Appendix C

Biographical Sketches of Workshop Speakers and Planning Committee Members

WORKSHOP SPEAKERS

Joan Bathon, M.D., is a rheumatologist, a professor of medicine, the chief of the Division of Rheumatology, and an advisory dean for clinician scientist faculty at the Columbia University Medical Center. Prior to that, she was the deputy director of rheumatology and the director of the Arthritis Center at Johns Hopkins Medical Institutions. Her career has focused on understanding the pathogenesis and functional consequences of inflammation in rheumatoid arthritis (RA). Her group is particularly interested in understanding the effects of chronic rheumatoid inflammation on the extra-articular phenotype of RA, as manifested by accelerated atherosclerosis, myocardial dysfunction, and adverse body composition. Her work has consistently been funded by the National Institutes of Health's (NIH's) National Institute of Arthritis and Musculoskeletal and Skin Diseases (NIAMS), the Rheumatology Research Foundation, and other sources. Dr. Bathon has also been the principal investigator or co-investigator on many RA and osteoarthritis clinical trials, both industry and NIH sponsored. She has authored more than 200 scientific publications and book chapters. Dr. Bathon is currently a member of the NIAMS Advisory Council. She previously served as a standing member of both the NIH Arthritis, Connective Tissue, and Skin and the NIH-NIAMS Arthritis and Musculoskeletal and Skin Diseases Clinical Trials study sections. She is the past editor-in-chief of *Arthritis & Rheumatology*, a past member of the Food and Drug Administration Arthritis Advisory Committee, and a past member of the Board of Directors of the American College of Rheumatology. Her dedication to advancing the careers of women faculty and trainees is reflected by her past roles while at Johns Hopkins as the director of the dean's Office of Women in Science and Medicine, the co-chair of the Women's Leadership Council, and the chair of the Department of Medicine's Task Force on Academic Careers of Women in Medicine.

Jerome Bickenbach, Ph.D., LL.B., is a permanent visiting professor in the Department of Health Sciences and Medicine at the University of Lucerne and a professor in the Department of Philosophy and Faculties of Law and Medicine at Queen's University. He is the author of *Physical Disability and Social Policy* (1993) and the co-editor of *Introduction to Disability* (1998), *Disability and Culture: Universalism and Diversity* (2000), *A Seat at the Table: Persons with Disabilities and Policy Making* (2001), *Quality of Life and Human Difference* (2003), and numerous articles and chapters in disability studies, focusing on the nature of disability and disability law and policy. He is a content editor of Sage Publications' proposed 5-volume *Encyclopaedia of Disability*. Since 1995, he has been a consultant with the World Health Organization (WHO) working on the revision of the *International Classification of Impairments, Disabilities, and Handicaps* to the final draft leading to the *International Classification of Functioning, Disability and Health* (ICF). Professor Bickenbach has participated in nearly all revision activities, and continues to consult with WHO on ICF dissemination and international disability social policy. His research is in disability studies, using qualitative and quantitative research techniques within the paradigm of participatory action research. Most recently, his research includes disability quality of life and the disability critique, disability epidemiology, universal design and inclusion, modeling disability statistics for population health surveys, the relationship between disability and health, and the ethics and the application of ICF to monitoring the implementation of the United Nations Convention on the Rights of Persons with Disabilities. As a lawyer, Professor Bickenbach was a human rights litigator, specializing in antidiscrimination for persons with intellectual impairments and mental illness.

Daniel J. Clauw, M.D., is a professor of anesthesiology, medicine (rheumatology), and psychiatry at the University of Michigan. He attended undergraduate and medical school at the University of Michigan, and then did his internal medicine residency and rheumatology fellowships at Georgetown University, where he eventually held roles including the chief of rheumatology and the vice chair of medicine. While at Georgetown University he assembled an interdisciplinary team that began to study the central nervous system contributions to a number of chronic pain disorders, including fibromyalgia, interstitial cystitis, low back pain, and Gulf War illnesses. This group of investigators, the Chronic Pain and Fatigue Research Center, moved to the University of Michigan in 2002. In addition to bringing this group to the University of Michigan, Dr. Clauw was also asked to lead the clinical research infrastructure serving the University of Michigan at that time. With strong support from University of Michigan leadership he helped expand clinical and translational research infrastructure dramatically, becoming the first assistant and then associate dean for clinical research (through 2009). He was also the first principal investigator (PI) of the University of Michigan Clinical and Translational Sciences Award and the founding director of the unit at Michigan that supports translational research—the Michigan Institute for Clinical and Health Research. He currently is co-PI of three National Institutes of Health center grants studying the mechanisms underlying chronic pain in urological and musculoskeletal disorders and is an active mentor of clinical and pain researchers.

Judith A. Cook, Ph.D., is an internationally recognized authority on mental health services research, specifically the study of clinical and rehabilitation outcomes of children and adults receiving community-based care. She directs a federally funded research center along with numerous grants focused on intervention science and psychiatric epidemiology. She designs and implements innovative programs to enhance mental health and behavioral health of vulnerable populations. She works with federal, state, and local authorities on behavioral health service system redesign and alternative financing strategies. Her recent work focuses on randomized controlled trials of evidence-based practice treatments for serious mental illness and outcomes of individuals with co-occurring mental illness and chronic medical conditions. She consults with federal agencies including the National Institutes of Health, the Social Security Administration, the Department of Labor, the Government Accountability Office, the Substance Abuse and Mental Health Services Administration, and the Department of Veterans Affairs. She is currently the principal investigator for the first national study of the prevalence of psychiatric and substance use disorders among women living with HIV/AIDS. She was a member of the National Institute of Mental Health Study Section on Mental Health Services in Specialty Settings from 2006 to 2009.

Amit Etkin, M.D., Ph.D., is the founder, the chief executive officer, and the chairman of Alto Neuroscience, as well as a professor in the Department of Psychiatry and Behavioral Sciences at Stanford University and a member of the Wu Tsai Neuroscience Institute at Stanford University.

He has received multiple awards, most notably the National Institutes of Health Director's Pioneer Award in 2017, for groundbreaking work in clinical psychiatry and neuroscience. Dr. Etkin is trained as both as a neuroscientist and a psychiatrist, with scientific experience ranging from molecular biology through machine learning and human clinical trials. The overarching aim of Dr. Etkin's work has been understanding the neural basis of emotional disorders and their treatment, and leveraging this knowledge to better understand how the brain works and to develop novel treatment interventions. Alto Neuroscience builds on this work in order to advance precision psychiatry with respect to actionable, real-world, clinical, and commercial outcomes.

Philip D. Harvey, Ph.D., is the Leonard M. Miller Professor of Psychiatry and a Veterans Affairs (VA) senior health scientist. He is the author of more than 1,000 scientific papers and abstracts and he has written more than 60 book chapters. He has been designated annually by Thompson-Reuters since 2010 as being in the top 1 percent of all mental health researchers in citations. He has received a number of awards, including the first systemic inflammatory response syndrome Clinical Scientist Distinguished Contributions award in 2012, the 2014 Alexander Gralnick Schizophrenia Research award from the American Psychiatric Foundation, the 2014 VA John Blair Barnwell award, and he will receive the Stanley Dean Award from the American College of Psychiatrists in 2021. He has received continuous federal funding since 1985. His research has focused on cognition and everyday functioning across neuropsychiatric conditions, with a special focus on severe mental illness. His research has also recently focused on technology in mental health and aging, including novel assessment strategies using ecological momentary assessment and various passive measurement strategies and technology-based interventions.

Kristi L. Kirschner, M.D., is a clinical professor in the University of Illinois College of Medicine (UICOM) Department of Medical Education, with a secondary appointment in the Department of Neurology and Rehabilitation. She is currently the subtheme leader for health humanities for the UICOM curriculum taskforce and overseeing the development and enhancement of the health humanities programs within the University of Illinois College of Medicine. Dr. Kirschner's academic interests include medical humanities and bioethics with a particular focus on disability issues and marginalized populations; the training of health care professionals about health humanities, bioethics, and disability; and health care access for people with disabilities, including reproductive health services. She also is an adjunct faculty member in the Department of Disabilities and Human Development at UIC where she worked with Carol Gill,

Ph.D., and Teresa Savage Ph.D., RN, to create the Certificate in Disability Ethics in 2003. As background, she is a physician specializing in physical medicine and rehabilitation with particular interest in the needs of patients with complex neurological disabilities, including adults with spina bifida, neuromuscular diseases, and cerebral palsy.

Virginia Byers Kraus, M.D., Ph.D., is a professor of medicine, pathology, and orthopedic surgery, and a faculty member of the Duke Molecular Physiology Institute in the Duke University School of Medicine. She is a practicing rheumatologist with 20 years of experience in osteoarthritis (OA) research. Dr. Kraus is the past president of the Osteoarthritis Research Society International (OARSI)—the premier organization focused on the prevention and treatment of OA through the promotion and presentation of research, education, and the worldwide dissemination of new knowledge. In 2019, she was elected to the Association of American Physicians and awarded the Lifetime Achievement Award from OARSI. She is the co-principal investigator of the OARSI/Foundation for the National Institutes of Health Osteoarthritis Biomarkers Consortium Project, which advances the validation and qualification of biomarkers for OA diagnosis, prognosis, and clinical trials. She also directs the Duke Biomarkers Shared Resource under the management of Janet Huebner. This facility assists investigators with the design and implementation of molecular and protein assays to evaluate biochemical and inflammatory markers. Dr. Kraus is also the director of the molecular measures core in the Center for the Study of Aging and Human Development. This has led to a long-time collaboration of the Kraus lab with the Stedman Nutrition Center that has culminated in the housing of these labs under the Duke Molecular Physiology Institute.

Jeffrey A. Lieberman, M.D., is the Lawrence C. Kolb Professor and the chairman of the Department of Psychiatry at the Columbia University College of Physicians and Surgeons; the director of the New York State Psychiatric Institute; and the psychiatrist-in-chief at the Columbia University Medical Center of the New York-Presbyterian Hospital. The Columbia University Department of Psychiatry is among the top ranked in the nation in psychiatric research funding from the National Institutes of Health and for psychiatry in the *U.S. News & World Report* Best Hospital rankings. Dr. Lieberman's work at Columbia University has advanced the understanding of the neurobiology and the treatment of schizophrenia and related psychotic disorders and led to the transformative mental health care strategy for the early detection and prevention of schizophrenia. He has authored or co-authored more than 600 articles published in scientific literature and wrote or edited 11 books on mental illness, psychopharmacology, and psychiatry. In recognition of this work, he has received many national and international honors and awards, and in 2000 he was elected to the National Academy of Medicine and in 2013 as the president of the American Psychiatric Association. More recently, Dr. Lieberman's work has extended into public policy and advocacy for enhancing awareness of mental illness and improving mental health care, as well as reducing the stigma associated with mental illness. In this context, Dr. Lieberman has actively contributed to government policy and federal legislation, including the Mental Health Parity and Addiction Equity Act, the Patient Protection and Affordable Care Act, and the Helping Families in Mental Health Crisis Act, and he is a visible spokesperson to the media on mental illness and psychiatry. This motivated him to write the critically acclaimed book *Shrinks: The Untold Story of Psychiatry* and deliver a TED talk on stigma and mental illness.

Joseph P. Menetski, Ph.D., is the associate vice president of research partnerships and the director of the Biomarkers Consortium at the Foundation for the National Institutes of Health. Dr. Menetski received his Ph.D. from the Northwestern University Medical School with Dr. Stephen Kowalczykowski and completed his postdoctoral training at the Laboratory of Molecular Biology at the National Institutes of Health's National Institute of Diabetes and Digestive and Kidney Diseases with Dr. Martin Gellert. He then started his career in industry in 1993 in the Immunopathology Department at Parke-Davis (later Pfizer), where he established a discovery research program in cellular inflammation that eventually transitioned to the molecular study of osteoarthritis (OA). Dr. Menetski moved to Merck in 2004. His first position was in the Department of Immunology where he was involved in the OA new targets and biomarker program. While at Merck he was a member of the Molecular Profiling group, the Knowledge Discovery and Knowledge Management group, and finally a director in Global Competitive Intelligence. Over the years, he has been a key contributor to many basic research and clinical programs in the areas of arthritis, sarcopenia, osteoporosis, and asthma. He has served as a core research team member on several external basic research projects for the identification of new targets and molecular biomarkers. His industry research and development experiences include target identification, compound selection, translational biomarker identification, clinical study design and analysis, and external scientific collaborations. In the commercial space, he has been intimately involved in opportunity and asset identification and qualification, and in assessing the competitive landscape of disease areas that he is supporting. During this time, he has been recognized by multiple research and development awards for his contributions.

Andrew Peterson, Ph.D., is an assistant professor in the Institute for Philosophy and Public Policy at George Mason University, an affiliate researcher at the University of Pennsylvania Memory Center, a guest researcher at the National Institutes of Health's Department of Bioethics, and a Greenwall Faculty Scholar. Previously, he was a Crest Fellow at the Potomac Institute for Policy Studies in Washington, DC, and a Vanier Canada Graduate Scholar (CGS) in the Rotman Institute of Philosophy and the Brain and Mind Institute at the University of Western Ontario, Canada. Dr. Peterson's research centers on bioethics and the philosophy of neuroscience, with specialization in ethical and epistemological issues related to the scientific study of consciousness. This work has been funded by the National Institute on Aging, the Vanier CGS program, the Canadian Institutes for Health Research, and The Greenwall Foundation.

Gwendolyn Sowa, M.D., Ph.D., is the Endowed Professor and the chair of the Department of Physical Medicine and Rehabilitation at the University of Pittsburgh and University of Pittsburgh Medical Center (UPMC). Dr. Sowa also serves as the co-director of the Ferguson Laboratory for Orthopaedic and Spine Research and the medical director of UPMC Total Care-Musculoskeletal Health. She holds joint appointments in the Departments of Orthopaedic Surgery and Bioengineering. Dr. Sowa completed her Ph.D. in biochemistry and M.D. at the University of Wisconsin–Madison and her physical medicine and rehabilitation residency at the Rehabilitation Institute of Chicago at Northwestern University. She has served as a clinician scientist in the Department of Physical Medicine and Rehabilitation for more than 15 years, where she has been active in developing new models of care for patients with low back pain. As the co-director of the Ferguson Laboratory, which has a rich history in musculoskeletal research, she leads a diverse group of scientists, including engineers, physiatrists, molecular biologists, orthopedic surgeons, and neurosurgeons working together to develop innovative and individualized treatments for spine conditions and low back pain. The ultimate goal of her research program is to apply the growing knowledge of the biology and mechanobiology of the spine to the development of biomarkers to facilitate precision medicine approaches for low back pain treatment.

Madhukar H. Trivedi, M.D., is a professor in the Department of Psychiatry at the University of Texas (UT) Southwestern Medical Center. He serves as the chief of the Division of Mood Disorders and the founding director of the Center for Depression Research and Clinical Care, where he holds the Betty Jo Hay Distinguished Chair in Mental Health and the Julie K. Hersh Chair for Depression Research and Clinical Care. He specializes in treating depression. Dr. Trivedi is an internationally recognized translational researcher focusing on developing and validating biosignatures of depression. He also conducts research on pharmacological, psychosocial, and nonpharmacological treatments for depression. Dr. Trivedi has authored more than 500 peer-reviewed research publications and he is currently the president of the American Society of Clinical Psychopharmacology. Dr. Trivedi earned his medical degree at Baroda Medical College in India, where he also completed a residency in psychiatry. He performed a second residency in psychiatry at Henry Ford Hospital in Detroit, Michigan, and received advanced training in functional brain imaging and psychopharmacology through a research fellowship at UT Southwestern.

Amy K. Wagner, M.D., is a tenured professor, the vice-chair of faculty development, and the Endowed Chair for Translational Research in the Department of Physical Medicine and Rehabilitation at the University of Pittsburgh and University of Pittsburgh Medical Center (UPMC). She holds a secondary appointment in the Department of Neuroscience and the Clinical Science and Research Institute. She is also the associate director for rehabilitation research at the Safar Center for Resuscitation Research and directs UPMC's Clinical Brain Injury Medicine Fellowship. Dr. Wagner's research program uses biomarkers as tools for developing and optimizing personalized treatments and outcomes for individuals with disability, particularly with traumatic brain injury (TBI) and with cardiac arrest. Dr. Wagner's research focus includes the TBI Rehabilomics Research Model, identifying biomarkers relevant for assessing pathology and prognosis as well as for assessing clinical risk and use in clinical decision making. Her experimental research also focuses on how agents commonly used during rehabilitation impact recovery. Her experimental research also focuses on the neurobiology of neuroplasticity and recovery after TBI, immunotherapies after neurological injury, and how commonly used therapeutic agents impact neurobiological and neurobehavioral processes associated with neuroplasticity and recovery. She is especially focused on dopaminergic systems and brain injury recovery, and her experimental TBI work also includes the study of rehabilitation relevant cognitive training paradigms to better understand the substrates and mechanisms of learning and memory recovery. She also conducts large database work identifying risk factors for complications after brain injury such as epilepsy and mental health disorders and development risk/prognostic models for these complications after TBI.

Mark Warshawsky, Ph.D., is the deputy commissioner for retirement and disability policy at the Social Security Administration. He is in charge of a policy, research, and administration component (about 520 employees);

identifying issues; assuring quality; responsiveness of policy development; analysis and data for agency leadership; and the administration. In particular, he is leading efforts to modernize the disability programs and to improve the vehicles that educate the public on program features. His interests include social security, employer-sponsored pension and retirement programs, financial planning, health and long-term care financing, public finance, and macroeconomics. He has testified before Congress and administrative agencies many times, and was recently a senior research fellow at the Mercatus Center of George Mason University, as well as a visiting scholar at the Massachusetts Institute of Technology Golub Center for Finance and Policy. Dr. Warshawsky is the author of more than 150 published articles and 4 books. From 2006 to 2013, he was the director of retirement research at Towers Watson, a global human capital consulting firm. Dr. Warshawsky was a member of the Social Security Advisory Board from 2006 through 2012 and was the vice chairman of the Federal Commission on Long-Term Care in 2013. From 2004 to 2006, Dr. Warshawsky served as the assistant secretary for economic policy at the Department of the Treasury, playing a key role in the development of the Pension Protection Act of 2006. He is the inventor of the life care annuity, a product integrating the immediate life annuity and long-term care insurance benefits, and a developer of planning software. Dr. Warshawsky has held senior-level positions at the Federal Reserve Board, the Internal Revenue Service, and the Teachers Insurance and Annuity Association-College Retirement Equities Fund. He received a Ph.D. in economics from Harvard University and a B.A. with the highest distinction from Northwestern University.

PLANNING COMMITTEE

Sara Rosenbaum, J.D. (*Chair*), is the Harold and Jane Hirsh Professor of Health Law and Policy and the founding chair of the Department of Health Policy at the Milken Institute School of Public Health at The George Washington University. She also holds professorships in the Trachtenberg School of Public Policy and Public Administration and the Schools of Law and Medicine and Health Sciences. A graduate of Wesleyan University and Boston University Law School, Professor Rosenbaum has devoted her career to issues of health justice for populations who are medically underserved as a result of race, poverty, disability, or cultural exclusion. An honored teacher and scholar, a highly popular speaker, and a widely read writer on many aspects of health law and policy, Professor Rosenbaum has emphasized public engagement as a core element of her professional life, providing public service to six presidential administrations and 19 Congresses. She is best known for her work on national health reform, Medicaid and private insurance, Medicaid managed care, health care access for medically underserved communities and populations, and civil rights and health care.

Linda S. Brady, Ph.D., serves as the director of the Division of Neuroscience and Basic Behavioral Science at the National Institute of Mental Health (NIMH). In this role, she provides scientific, programmatic, and administrative leadership for an extramural research program portfolio in basic neuroscience to support NIMH's mission of transforming the understanding and treatment of mental illnesses. Dr. Brady has directed programs in neuropharmacology, drug discovery, and clinical therapeutics and organized consortia focused on ways to accelerate the development and clinical application of radiotracers in clinical research. She has provided leadership for many programs, including Development and Application of Positron Emission Tomography and Single Photon Emission Computed Tomography Imaging Ligands as Biomarkers for Drug Discovery and for Pathophysiological Studies of Central Nervous System Disorders, the National Cooperative Drug/Device Discovery/Development Groups for the Treatment of Mental Disorders, and First in Human and Early Stage Clinical Trials of Novel Investigational Drugs or Devices for Psychiatric Disorders. Dr. Brady serves as the co-chair of the Neuroscience Steering Committee for the Biomarkers Consortium, a public–private research partnership of the Foundation for the National Institutes of Health that focuses on discovery, development, and qualification of biological markers to support drug development, preventive medicine, and medical diagnostics. From 2004 to 2013, she was the co-leader of the Molecular Libraries and Imaging Program, a trans-National Institutes of Health (NIH) Common Fund initiative to provide biomedical researchers access to small organic molecules that can be used as chemical probes to study the functions of genes, cells, and biochemical pathways in health and disease. Dr. Brady was trained in pharmacology and neuroscience. She completed her Ph.D. at the Emory University School of Medicine, followed by postdoctoral work and research positions at the Uniformed Services University of the Health Sciences and the NIMH Intramural Research Program. She is the author of more than 70 peer-reviewed scientific publications and is a member of the Society for Neuroscience and a Fellow in the American College of Neuropsychopharmacology. Dr. Brady has received NIH Director awards and NIH Merit awards in recognition of her activities in biomarker development and drug development for mental disorders.

Betty Diamond, M.D., graduated with a B.A. from Harvard University and an M.D. from Harvard Medical School. She performed a residency in internal medicine at the Columbia Presbyterian Medical Center and received postdoctoral training in immunology at the Albert Einstein College of Medicine. Dr. Diamond has headed the rheumatology divisions at the Albert Einstein School of Medicine and the Columbia University Medical Center. She also directed the Medical Scientist Training Program at the Albert Einstein School of Medicine for many years. She is currently the head of the Center for Autoimmune, Musculoskeletal and Hematopoietic Diseases at the Feinstein Institutes for Medical Research and the director of the Ph.D. and M.D./Ph.D. programs of the Donald and Barbara Zucker School of Medicine at Hofstra/Northwell. A former president of the American Association of Immunology, Dr. Diamond has also served on the Board of Directors of the American College of Rheumatology and the Scientific Council of the National Institute of Arthritis and Musculoskeletal and Skin Diseases. Dr. Diamond is a fellow of the American Association for the Advancement of Science and a member of the National Academy of Medicine.

Sarah E. Morris, Ph.D., is the chief of the Adult Psychopathology and Psychosocial Interventions Research Branch of the National Institute of Mental Health (NIMH) Division of Translational Research and associate head of the Research Domain Criteria (RDoC) Unit. Dr. Morris earned her B.A. in psychology from Scripps College and her M.A. and Ph.D. from the University of California, Los Angeles, where she studied the processing of emotional and auditory stimuli and error detection in schizophrenia using psychophysiological methods. She completed a clinical internship at the West Los Angeles Veterans Affairs (VA) Medical Center and a postdoctoral fellowship at the Mental Illness Research, Education and Clinical Center (MIRECC) at the Baltimore VA Medical Center. Following her fellowship, Dr. Morris joined the faculty in the Department of Psychiatry at the University of Maryland School of Medicine and continued as an investigator at the MIRECC. She also served as the director of the VA Maryland Health Care System/University of Maryland Baltimore Psychology Internship Consortium. Her research has focused on learning, reward processing, and self-monitoring in schizophrenia using event-related brain potentials and on remediation of cognitive deficits in schizophrenia. She joined NIMH in 2010 as a program officer for the schizophrenia-spectrum disorders program and now leads a branch that manages inquiries, grant applications, and funded grants focused on translational research in adult psychopathology and co-leads the RDoC effort to explore novel methods to classify mental disorders.

Ralph Nitkin, Ph.D., is the deputy director for the National Institute of Child Health and Human Development's (NICHD's) National Center for Medical Rehabilitation Research (NCMRR). For the past 30 years, he has worked as a science administrator at NICHD, first in intellectual and developmental disabilities and, for the past 20 years, in medical rehabilitation. Within NCMRR, Dr. Nitkin is particularly involved with research on the fundamental mechanisms and substrate of rehabilitation, including neuroplasticity, physiology, exercise, and other adaptive changes. He also leads efforts on NCMRR rehabilitation research infrastructure networks (now the Medical Rehabilitation Research Resource Network), the annual Training in Grantsmanship for Rehabilitation Research grant-writing workshop, and special career development networks for clinical neurorehabilitation, for physical/occupational therapists, and, more recently, for rehabilitation engineers. In addition to his NCMRR work, Dr. Nitkin has helped promote National Institutes of Health research initiatives in diverse areas such as genomic factors that affect rehabilitation outcomes, promotion of exercise and diet in children with disabilities, clinical trial design in rehabilitation, technologies for healthy independent living, and research workforce diversity. Dr. Nitkin received his undergraduate and master's degrees in biological sciences from the Massachusetts Institute of Technology and his Ph.D. in cellular neurobiology from the University of California, San Diego. His postdoctoral studies at Stanford University and later work as an assistant professor at Rutgers University focused on the cellular and molecular basis of nerve—muscle synapse formation.

Patricia M. Owens has been a member of the National Academy of Social Insurance since 1993. She currently serves on the Board of Directors and recently accepted the position of chair to the Development Committee. Ms. Owens consults internationally on disability policy in both public and private sectors. Previously, she was the senior disability advisor and the vice president at UNUM Life Insurance Company. Before that, she was the vice president of group and individual underwriting at the Paul Revere Insurance Group. From 1982 to 1986, Ms. Owens served as the associate U.S. commissioner for disability at the Social Security Administration (SSA). While at SSA, she received the Health and Human Services Distinguished Leadership Award and a Social Security Commissioner's Public Service Citation. She was a Switzer Fellow and author of the National Rehabilitation Association and was a member of the Notch Commission. She served on the National Academy of Social Insurance Disability Policy Panel. Ms. Owens has written a number of reports and monographs on disability-related issues and legislation.

Sarah Ruiz, Ph.D., is an associate director of the Office of Research Sciences at the National Institute on Disability, Independent Living, and Rehabilitation Research. Her current research focuses on evidence-based programs and practices for individuals aging with long-term disability. She has more than 15 years of experience designing and analyzing research studies on health outcomes for older adults and people with disabilities, with extensive experience working on projects at the federal, state, and local level. In her past role at NORC at the University of Chicago, she led large-scale program evaluation efforts to understand health care innovation for older adults and people with disabilities under the Patient Protection and Affordable Care Act. Dr. Ruiz has also held leadership positions in the nonprofit and private sectors. She served as the research director for the National Self-Management Alliance, a public–private partnership to scale chronic disease self-management interventions at the National Council on Aging that arose from the Department of Health and Human Services' Strategic Framework on Multiple Chronic Conditions. Dr. Ruiz was previously a research associate at the RAND Corporation and IMPAQ International, where she managed and oversaw projects on health policy, long-term care, and evidence-based programs and services for older adults. She holds a Ph.D. in gerontology from the University of Southern California.

Ira Shoulson, M.D., is a professor of neurology, pharmacology, and human science and the director of the Program for Regulatory Science and Medicine at Georgetown University in Washington, DC. From 1990 until 2011, Dr. Shoulson was the Louis C. Lasagna Professor of Experimental Therapeutics and a professor of neurology, pharmacology, and medicine at the University of Rochester School of Medicine and Dentistry in Rochester, New York, where he currently holds adjunct appointments as a professor of neurology, pharmacology, and physiology. Dr. Shoulson founded the Parkinson Study Group in 1985 and the Huntington Study Group in 1994—international academic consortia devoted to research and development of treatments for Parkinson's disease, Huntington's disease, and related neurodegenerative and neurogenetic disorders. He was a key investigator in the United States–Venezuela Collaborative Huntington's Disease Project, which identified the gene responsible for this fatal hereditary disorder. Dr. Shoulson has served as the principal investigator of the National Institutes of Health–sponsored trials "Deprenyl and Tocopherol Antioxidative Therapy of Parkinsonism," the "Prospective Huntington at Risk Observational Study," and in the leadership of more than 35 other multi-center clinical research studies. He played an instrumental role in the development of 10 new drugs for neurological disorders, including seven for Parkinson's disease (selegiline, lazabemide, pramipexole, entacapone, clozapine, rasagiline, rotigitine), two for Huntington's disease (tetrabenazine, dutetetrabenazine), and one for attention deficit disorder (Concerta). He was formerly a health policy fellow in the U.S. Senate, a member of the National Institute of Neurological Disorders and Stroke Council, and the president of the American Society for Experimental NeuroTherapeutics. He is currently a principal investigator of the Food and Drug Administration-Georgetown University Collaborating Center of Excellence in Regulatory Science and Innovation (CERSI–FD004319), the associate editor of *JAMA Neurology,* and an active elected member of the National Academy of Medicine. He has authored more than 310 scientific reports.

Robert B. Wallace, M.D., M.Sc., is interested in the occurrence and prevention of chronic illnesses and disabilities in older persons. He has worked in the areas of prevention of coronary artery disease, stroke, osteoarthritis, dementia, osteoporotic fractures, and various common cancers. In addition to the Health and Retirement Study, he has participated in trials of the prevention of disease, disability and falls, and in the common chronic conditions of postmenopausal women. He has been an investigator or consultant for other cohort studies of older persons, including the National Health and Aging Trends Study; the English Longitudinal Study of Ageing; the National Social Life, Health, and Aging Project; the Mexican Health and Aging Study; and the Hispanic Established Populations for the Epidemiologic Study of the Elderly.